Common Sense Biblical Approach to Health and Fitness

TIM FRADY

DEDICATION

I just want to take the opportunity to thank God first and foremost, and my wife Teresa for helping me put this book together.

DISCLAIMER

The views and information presented in this book are for informational purposes only and are not meant to take the place of the advice of a qualified medical professional or doctor. Always seek the advice of a medical professional before making changes to your diet, exercise, or other health regimes.

CONTENTS

ACKNOWLEDGMENTS

My wife and I really enjoy the gym where we work out, Foust's Family Fitness. We appreciate the hard work Paul Faust does in creating a great friendly work out environment.

I'd like to thank our pastor at Mount Pisgah Baptist Church, Garvan Walls, who has inspired me with his messages filled with spiritual wisdom and just plain old great common sense preaching.

I also am glad to have a good friend like Brad Parish who gave me the idea to write this book in the first place.

Of course, I have to thank my wife for putting up with me and giving me encouragement. She also helped with editing, and added a lot to the book in general.

Come by and visit our website hip2bfit.com for daily health and fitness news and articles.

1 PURPOSE OF THIS BOOK

I think it's important to put into perspective the reasons for the book you the reader have in your hands right now. First of all, let me say that my goal in writing this book is definitely not to say that being overweight is a sin, or that somehow the number of push-ups a person can do somehow makes them more spiritual or closer to God in any way. But let me say that while being overweight may not be a sin, gluttony is.

I hope to enable you the reader to not only have a greater understanding of health and fitness concepts, but to show how living healthy is indeed a spiritual concept as well. In fact, I had to write this book from a Biblical world view to be honest to my own personal outlook of health and fitness. I can't imagine a complete view of health and fitness that divorced itself from the spiritual. While it is possible to be healthy and not be a Christian of course, I do not believe it is possible to live as healthy as God intended us to without a close relationship to Jesus Christ and without following the simple concepts the Bible teaches us. Sin and failure to follow God's word really does have a negative effect on health.

What has motivated me to write this book is the growing tendency for great Christian people to simply dismiss their focus on health as being worldly and not worthy of their attention. God does take care of his children of course, but He doesn't always erase the consequences of our foolish lifestyle choices. Think of all the wonderful preachers, teachers, singers, church members, missionaries, and Christians from every walk of life whose life or ministry may have been cut short because of an overindulgence in junk food, a lack of understanding of the dangers of too much sugar, and too little exercise and physical activity.

As sure as putting sugar in a gas tank will cause your car to sputter, putting too much into your body will do the same. Would you pour a bag of sugar into the church bus expecting God to make the engine run fine? Even though we may be doing the Lord's will, I think He still expects us to use common sense when it comes to what we put into our bodies.

No one has a right to make judgments based on a person's appearance or weight, but what I hope this book will do is encourage you the reader to take an honest look at your eating habits and activity level to see if there is room for improvement, so you don't cheat yourself out of years of life and activity.

If you are consistently gaining fat every month, then odds are you aren't eating properly. Some weight gain as we get older is natural, but excessive weight gain is usually a sign that something is wrong somewhere. If it's not in your diet or activity level then it's time to see a doctor and find out what maybe wrong with you physically. It could be something like a thyroid disorder, for instance.

The truth is, we could all benefit from eating natural foods and giving up sugary, processed foods. It doesn't matter if you are a star athlete or just someone looking to shed a few pounds. Eating fruits, vegetables, and healthy meats can make a vast improvement in a person's health and fat level over time, including athletic performance. It's not nearly as difficult as some believe to make long lasting health changes that the average person can live with. I hope and pray that more people will give it a try and see how living healthy can vastly improve their own quality of life.

Along the way of discussing healthy lifestyle choices we'll investigate how following the health principles in the Bible can make you healthier and happier. This isn't a health and wealth book by the way. There is no magic bullet. Asking God to lose forty pounds and/or to add ten pounds of muscle isn't going to work without being willing to make the changes or do the work involved.

I do encourage you to pray about meeting health goals, though. Just don't be surprised to find out that it means God gives you the strength you need to make some changes in your life. Starting new healthy habits for the first time is sometimes the hardest part. Once you get into a good habit for a while it becomes a part of your daily routine. God has given us lots of great healthy foods; all you have to do is start eating them and stop eating the unhealthy processed man made foods.

Christians should be the healthiest people on the planet, and in truth we do have a lot of health advantages over others who don't claim to be Christians. For instance, we have a great outlet through prayer to God to cast our burdens and cares down which is a great stress reliever. I firmly believe stress can cause more damage to a person's health than even smoking and eating sugar all day long. That being said, though, the obesity epidemic brought on by sugar consumption has wrought mass destruction on the health of Christians and non-Christians alike. Although I do believe it has been hitting the general public harder than those that regularly attend church. The reason being that those that seek after God are less likely to take in food to satisfy their inner needs. Those in the world are desperately trying to fill their spiritual needs with anything they can, and most of the time these days that becomes foods with high sugar content. Still, I think a lot of Christians may be using food to replace God in their lives and may not even be aware that they are committing a sin of idolatry as well as gluttony. Baptists, of whom I am one, especially love to eat. For the most part, Baptists don't like to look at eating food as being an actual sin, but anything can be a sin if it takes the place of God in our lives.

Today food has become the new drug of choice when we feel stressed, worried, or discouraged. I can understand up to a point the temptation to turn to food in times of stress, but those are times we need to turn to God in prayer, and spend time working on solving the actual problem instead of eating junk food.

There are so many ways to go about attacking the food addiction. Buying healthy food to take the place of unhealthy food is the first step. Taking the time to prepare a healthy meal is time you aren't eating fast but dangerous junk food. Think about all the things you miss out on in life that junk food can deny you. Obesity and diabetes can rob you of years of life and enjoyable activities you can take part in.

We are all guilty of putting too much emphasis on food. Since eating is necessary to survive, and obviously God meant for us to eat, we have a hard time realizing that overeating can be as big a sin as smoking or getting intoxicated with alcohol. By seeking that sugar fix anytime we feel depressed, we are no better than the junkie, or the alcoholic. Processed sugar is a drug, and I can prove it to you. We'll talk more later about what the Bible says about gluttony.

Look around you on your next trip to the grocery store and you'll see a lot of people who are not just overweight, but morbidly obese. It's really heartbreaking when you think of how many people have their lives turned upside down by sugar and junky processed foods. The statistics show that more and more Americans are getting there. They are hooked on the sugar drug, and they will not stop taking it even if it kills them, and it just might.

Part of this book will take more time to look at exactly what is wrong with eating too much sugar, but the short version is that it triggers insulin, causes inflammation, doesn't satisfy your nutritional needs, and ultimately makes a person steadily gain weight from week to week. Processed sugary foods are poison to your body.

The addiction to sugar is real. Why else would a human being continue to devour processed garbage day in and day out as their body becomes so unhealthy that even the task of walking becomes a hardship. I'm talking about people that could be active, healthy individuals, but they can't stop eating the wrong kinds of foods. They might tell you it's just a choice or that it just tastes too good to stop, but is it rational to drink or eat poison because it tastes good?

But don't be too discouraged, food can be enjoyed without hurting your health or having an unnatural addiction. People don't realize just how good and tasty healthy foods can be. Sure, these foods may take a little more effort to prepare, but, in the long run, it's a lot easier than being hooked up to life support.

Probably, one of the things that Has inspired me the most to write this book has been the long list of prayer requests our church gets every day. So many people seem to get sick and pass away that, while one realizes that a person's passing or sickness is in the hands of God, I still wonder and hope that by utilizing diet and fitness knowledge and the wisdom in God's Word, perhaps more people might prolong their lives, or at the very least, avoid many illnesses during their lives.

Cancer and heart disease are two of the biggest killers in America, and yet there are so many ways to fight these two diseases via avoiding bad food and eating the real food that God provided for us and intended for us to eat. As I will discuss further later, fruits, vegetables, and spices are known for their anti-cancer properties and nutrients, while, on the other hand, fast food, processed sugar snacks, and soft drinks all may cause cancer or at least are suspected of creating a greater risk for cancer. Just watching what you eat can make a huge difference in the fight against disease, and, by taking the principles found in the Bible concerning issues that cause stress in our lives, you have two huge weapons in your arsenal against disease.

Add to that a helping of vitamin D whenever a few minutes of sun exposure is possible, plus exercise, and eventually the risks of diseases starts to shrink. There is no way to totally wipe out heart disease and cancer, but I think it could make a huge impact in the church if health issues were focused on a little more. Let's understand that God is the Great Physician and yes we need to pray for healing and help in our daily lives, but I believe that God has given us many prescriptions for our ailments via all the many healthy foods He created, and the principles in His Word that really do the physical body good as well as the spiritual.

When the spiritual body is healthy, the physical body tends to follow, but again we need a complete picture that creates balance in our physical lives by eating healthy and exercising. For example man cannot duplicate in supplement form the numerous amounts of nutrients and phytochemicals that are found in fruits and vegetables. While I take supplements myself, I know for a fact that no supplement is superior to what you can get in natural food that God created. It seems that the more man gets involved with his chemicals and additives the more harmful and less beneficial foods become.

There is complete harmony in science, health, and God's Word. You will not find commands from God in the Bible that are unhealthy for you. Refusing to lie, cheat, steal, or take God's name in vain will not hurt your health, but, in fact, as we discuss later, sins, especially ones that lead to anger and stress can and will cause harm to your body.

I'm reminded of a old joke our pastor, I believe, has told in the past. There was a man trapped in a flood that prayed for rescue. A raft came by and he refused to get on board, instead opting to wait for God's deliverance. Two boats go by, but he still refuses insisting on waiting on God. Finally, while on the rooftop of his home, as the water almost covers his home, a helicopter flies over, and still the man refuses to get on board. Later in heaven he asks St. Peter why he wasn't delivered from the flood, and St. Peter answers, "We sent you a raft, two boats, and a helicopter".

I think sometimes we are that way. God has made provisions for us but we just refuse to accept those provisions. It also reminds me of those that are lost that try to get to heaven on their own good works instead of relying on the provision that God has provided for us through the death, burial, and resurrection of Jesus, our Lord and Savior. Humanity is naturally stubborn. Sometimes it's not enough for us to have our needs met, we want them met the exact way we want, or we don't want it. Pride, another harmful, unhealthy sin seems to have a big part in that.

2 MY HEALTH AND FITNESS JOURNEY

I grew up in the 70's and 80's, back when kids drank cokes and ate lots of candy bars, but, at the same time, back then we were expected to go outside and play, ride bikes and be active. So being fat was never a problem for me back then, even though I ate fried chicken like it was going out of style.

In fact, I had the opposite problem. I was always too thin and small in general. This led to some issues on the playground when I was young. Kids love to pick on the little guy. So, as I got into my teens, I started getting interested in weight lifting to build my puny body into something a little more like my favorite action hero, Sylvester Stallone. The Rocky movies were my first introduction to the concept that a guy could literally build his body to look like he wanted. So I was able to get my hands on some cheap weights sometime in my very early teens. I worked out a lot, but never really saw much improvement. Of course, I knew nothing at all about eating healthy or how to train properly. My favorite meals were fried chicken, hamburgers, canned chili, and ice cream. It wasn't until I was about 16 years old that I started going to a local gym, and there I finally began to see some results.

My prime motivating factor was always my gym workout goals. Working out with goals in mind not only helps you move to where you want to be, it shows you where you are now. Testing yourself physically in a gym can let you see just where you are and what you need to do to make changes. Although you shouldn't try to directly compete with people that have been in the gym for years because that can lead to injuries, seeing where other people are at can be motivational and it helps give you an idea of where you should be.

Ultimately, my fitness goals now have a balanced approach. I want to be reasonably able to do a little bit of everything, whether it's running, jumping, being flexible, or lifting weights. Variety is important and it makes working out fun. Of course, now my workouts aren't just about being big and having lots of muscles. I've graduated to wanting the best of both worlds, that is, being healthy first and then using my fitness level as sort of a gauge of where I'm at and what I need to work on to keep me going in the direction of a healthy lifestyle.

Over the years, I've wrestled with smoking cigarettes, and took a few more years to ditch the soft drink addiction. I've learned a lot of lessons about how important diet is to overall health and fitness. As important as exercise is, you just can't do it all with exercise alone; it's not a "get out of jail free card". You can't smoke, or eat disease causing junk food and expect to be healthy or very effective in the gym no matter how hard you work out. It becomes more and more obvious the older you get that what you put into your tank is of the utmost importance.

I've seen 20-30 pounds of fat caused by junk food melt off my body just by changing my diet. It's definitely not that I work out harder, or that I eat that much less. In fact, I may eat more now than I ever have. I know it's possible, with the help of God, to give up any bad habit whether it's smoking or junk food.

I was raised on junk food, back when high fructose corn syrup was just getting started, and cokes were what I drank instead of water. Water was boring and tasteless to me when I was growing up. I wish someone had explained to me the dangers of sugar, and how much farther ahead I could have gotten with my workouts without it.

Hopefully, I can help people avoid the junk food trap I was in, and perhaps my experiences and research into health and fitness all these years can be a help or a blessing to others.

For the last few years I've ramped up my research into health and fitness and created a website, http://www.hip2bfit.com, that is centered around the steady stream of health news that is published almost every day. But, no matter what science discovers, in the end, it always backs up what common sense and the Bible have always told us about health. Eat healthy, be active, and avoid stress, which can be done by following the principles of the Bible, like loving others, avoiding anger, forgiving others, letting go of bitterness, and so on.

3 BIBLICAL HEALTH PRINCIPLES

The Bible strongly correlates obedience to God's commandments and longer life:

Proverbs 10:27
The fear of the LORD prolongeth days: but the years of the wicked shall be shortened .

Proverbs 3:1-2
1 My son, forget not my law; but let thine heart keep my commandments: 2 For length of days, and long life, and peace, shall they add to thee.

Exodus 20:12
Honour thy father and thy mother: that thy days may be long upon the land which the LORD thy God giveth thee.

Deuteronomy 30:20
That thou mayest love the LORD thy God, and that thou mayest obey his voice, and that thou mayest cleave unto him: for he is thy life, and the length of thy days: that thou mayest dwell in the land which the LORD sware unto thy fathers, to Abraham, to Isaac, and to Jacob, to give them.

It's remarkable how many Biblical principles affect health and longer life expectancy, like the need to work, being content, and not worrying. Take for instance the verse from Proverbs 17:22 that reads:

A merry heart doeth good like a medicine: but a broken spirit drieth the bones.

Research shows that laughter does the heart good, by expanding the linings of blood vessels and boosting blood flow.

In one study presented to the American Heart Association researchers found that people with heart disease were 40 percent less likely to laugh in various situations when compared to people of the same age who did not have heart disease. Part of the study asked participants questions like what you would do if someone spilled a drink on you. If the answer is laugh, or find it amusing, then you answered correctly on the side of health. People that find humor in situations, instead of finding reasons to fly off the handle, are less likely to have heart disease. So, here we find yet another correlation to Biblical principles like patience, being slow to anger, and not worrying. Further proof that, as the Bible teaches us, a merry heart is like medicine, thus, the opposite must be true for anger.

Did you know that mental stress is associated with impairment of the endothelium, the protective barrier lining our blood vessels? This can cause a series of inflammatory reactions that lead build-up in the coronary arteries, which can ultimately cause a heart attack.

The Bible doesn't teach us that we should never get angry. It teaches us to be slow to anger. Many times the Bible says God was angry at sin, but it also says in Psalm 145:8:

The LORD is gracious, and full of compassion; **slow to anger**, and of great mercy.

Proverbs 15:18
A wrathful man stirreth up strife. But he that is slow to anger appeaseth strife.

And in Proverbs 16:32
He that is slow to anger is better than the mighty; and he that ruleth his spirit than he that taketh a city.

There are other verses too that emphasize that God is slow to anger. The lesson then would be that we too should not react suddenly with anger. I don't think anyone would disagree that anger itself is not a healthy state.

Pride Verses Confidence

Proverbs 16:18 warns us against having a proud heart.

Pride goeth before destruction, and a haughty spirit before a fall.

I think one of the things that I've struggled with as a Christian is avoiding being filled with pride, and yet not being down on myself. There seems to be a fine line until you start to dissect the difference between the kind of pride I believe the Bible teaches against, and just have a health sense of confidence.

You need confidence to really do well in life, whether it's reaching a fitness goal, doing well at work, school, or any other pursuit. Wicked pride says, "I am self-sufficient". That kind of pride says that God is not needed. A person having that kind of pride is likely to feel that they are owed a living, love, or adoration simply because they exist. They do not feel the need to earn anything. They believe they should command respect above that of other human beings simply because they are who they are, by virtue of birth, as if they were born into royalty.

Confidence, on the other hand, says that I am capable of doing the same job, getting fit, earning a living, or making good grades just as much as the next person. That person sees what can be accomplished through hard work, but doesn't see themselves as being above the effort needed to accomplish their goals. They are willing to pray, work hard, eat right, study, exercise, or do whatever it takes to accomplish a goal. Confidence is about getting something done. Pride is feeling superior to other people. A lot of young people have this kind of pride these days. You can always tell when a man or woman has been told their entire life that they are God's gift to the human race. When confidence in ability switches to feelings of self-importance over and above others, you've gone too far.

When you think about it, someone with a prideful heart is least likely to put in the hard work in the gym to get into shape because a proud person may already see themselves as being better than those around them, regardless of their physical conditioning, or any other factors. The confident person sees a need in their life, whether its fitness or some other area, and seeks to reach that goal. You can also see how this could affect someone's spiritual condition, as someone filled with pride doesn't reach out to God, despite their need for a Saviour.

There are, of course, very hard working successful people that feel superior to others after a time. Sometimes we forget to thank God for the ability He gives us to work and to accomplish our goals, and we turn confidence into sinful pride. It's not working hard for money, or being fit that makes us filled with sinful pride, sometimes, it's after we achieve our goals we forget that the only difference between us and someone else is a lot of hard work and an answered prayer.

Don't let sinful pride cause you to believe you don't need to exercise to better yourself, and don't let a lack of confidence cause you to believe you can't accomplish anything that any other person can achieve. Aim your goals as far away as possible and work toward them. Even if you do fail to reach them, at least right away, you will have gone so much farther than you would have otherwise.

No one person is superior to anyone else. Some people may have better genes and be able to instantly grow their muscles an inch just by picking up a weight, while others struggle. But if you are physically able to lift a weight, or exercise, then you can be physically fit well beyond the average American these days. All it takes is a little hard work and a willingness to eat real food.

Here are just a few more verses against pride from the Bible:

Psalm 10:2
The wicked in his pride doth persecute the poor: let them be taken In the devices that they have imagined.

Psalm 10:4
The wicked, through the pride of his countenance, will not seek after God: God is not in all his thoughts.

Proverbs 11:2
When pride cometh, then cometh shame: but with the lowly is wisdom.

Proverbs 29:23
A man's pride shall bring him low: but honour shall uphold the humble in spirit.

Ezekiel 16:49
Behold, this was the iniquity of thy sister Sodom, pride, fullness of bread, and abundance of idleness was in her and in her daughters, neither did she strengthen the hand of the poor and needy.

Mark 7:22-23
22 Thefts, covetousness, wickedness, deceit, lasciviousness, an evil eye, blasphemy, pride, foolishness: 23 All these evil things come from within, and defile the man.

Psalm 101:5
Whoso privily slandereth his neighbour, him will I cut off: him that hath an high look and a proud heart will not I suffer .

And all of that is just a small portion of the verses that teach that pride is evil. Pride leads to anger and frustration. We take ourselves so seriously sometimes that we can't allow any infractions upon our person, or upon our pride, if you will. This leads to anger when a situation arises that makes us feel like someone has wronged us, no matter how small the infraction. Pride tends to cause us to blow things out of proportion. Anger leads to frustration, which leads back to negative effects on our health.

Long term anger has been linked to many health issues like high blood pressure, heart problems, skin problems, headaches, and problems with digestion. Those that have survived a heart attack, who remain stressed out, could be at risk for a fatal heart attack down the road.

And again we circle back to the Biblical principle of being slow to anger.

Ephesians 4:31
Let all bitterness, and wrath, and anger, and clamour, and evil speaking, be put away from you, with all malice:

Colossians 3:8
But now ye also put off all these; anger, wrath, malice, blasphemy, filthy communication out of your mouth.

Colossians 3:21
Fathers, provoke not your children to anger, lest they be discouraged.

Matthew 5:22
But I say unto you, That whosoever is angry with his brother without a cause shall be in danger of the judgment: and whosoever shall say to his brother, Raca, shall be in danger of the council: but whosoever shall say, Thou fool, shall be in danger of hell fire.

Titus 1:7
For a bishop must be blameless, as the steward of God; not selfwilled, not soon angry, not given to wine, no striker, not given to filthy lucre;

Again the idea is to be slow to anger. Flying off the handle at the slightest provocation will most likely hurt you a lot more than it will hurt the person you are angry with. They'll just think you're a jerk and go on their way while your arteries harden and you inch closer and closer to a heart attack. So think before you react. Taking time to think about whether or not your anger is justified, or if it's even worth getting angry over, can diffuse the inner time bomb inside.

So be careful when you find yourself getting angry over what that guy in front of you did in traffic. Remember, he doesn't know or care that you're angry. The only hope you have for revenge is that he'll see the angry expression on your face in his rearview mirror and become angry as well and have his arteries harden. Now you've just committed murder over a traffic nuisance. Was it worth it?

The Bible even offers some strategy in helping overcome a tense situation. Proverbs 15:1 says, "A soft answer turneth away wrath: but grievous words stir up anger". That's a good one to remember whether you are talking to your wife, your kids, or on the telephone discussing a bill or getting technical support. It works like this – you sense anger or frustration in the person that you are speaking with and your first inclination is to get angry back and feel proud, righteous indignation that this person deserves your wrath. The angrier you get with someone, the angrier they get with you, then you get even angrier with them, and on it goes until someone gets shot, has a heart attack, or a marriage ends in divorce.

It's a no win situation to think you can out anger someone and make them see the error of their ways. If you really want to convince someone that they've made a mistake, you have to do it kindly and patiently. Instead of getting angry, keep calm and speak gently, not showing anger or frustration. If you do this, what are the chances that the other person will be less likely to be angry in return?

Losing your temper can cost you friends too. Studies have shown that individuals who have good relationships with family and friends are healthier, but to do that you have be a good friend.

Proverbs 18:24
A man that hath friends must shew himself friendly: and there is a friend that sticketh closer than a brother.

Our emotional state deeply affects our health. There's no way around it. Our emotions are controlled, for the most part, not just by outward circumstances, but how we perceive those events in our mind's eye. Following biblical principles and behaving like Jesus, who only got angry when it was indeed an instance of a righteous cause, will go a long way toward helping us all be healthier. It seems that God's commandments aren't about stopping us from having fun, but go a long way toward keeping us alive longer.

Luke 3:14
And the soldiers likewise demanded of him, saying , And what shall we do ? And he said unto them, Do violence to no man, neither accuse any falsely; and be content with your wages

Philippians 4:11
Not that I speak in respect of want: for I have learned, in whatsoever state I am, therewith to be content.

1 Timothy 6:8
And having food and raiment let us be therewith content .

Hebrews 13:5
Let your conversation be without covetousness; and be content with such things as ye have: for he hath said, I will never leave thee, nor forsake thee.

Negative emotions have been linked to all diseases, including cancer. If a person has to deal with lots of stress, it's probable that that person may soon have some health issues to deal with as well. If, however, that person can manage to deal with their situations effectively without going into emotional overload, then it's possible they can skip the negative health consequences. Therefore, by acting on the Bible principle to be content in whatever state you are in, you are creating a stable emotional state that could greatly decrease your chances of diseases later on.

Also, good old activity, like exercise, is a great way to relieve stress, deal with anger, and help a person overcome the blues. Sitting around too much can lead to depression. God didn't make us to sit all day. Research shows people that sit all day, even at work, are more likely to have a cardiac event than someone who is at least somewhat active all day.

Cortisol and Stress

Another problem with stress is that it increases cortisol, a stress hormone produced by the adrenal glands in response to stress. Not getting enough sleep can increase cortisol along with everyday stress, and cortisol is one of the culprits responsible for giving us belly fat. It has been said that just 15 minutes a day set aside for relaxation can reduce cortisol levels. Interestingly enough, that also sounds like a good reason for Christians to set aside a few minutes for prayer and Bible study every day. Think about it. Prayer and Bible study in a quite environment is a great way to relax, and, at the same time you are slimming down your stomach and reducing harmful stress.

Consider Psalm 23:
1 The LORD is my shepherd; I shall not want. 2 He maketh me to lie down in green pastures: he leadeth me beside the still waters. 3 He restoreth my soul: he leadeth me in the paths of righteousness for

his name's sake. 4 Yea, though I walk through the valley of the shadow of death, I will fear no evil: for thou art with me; thy rod and thy staff they comfort me. 5 Thou preparest a table before me in the presence of mine enemies: thou anointest my head with oil; my cup runneth over. 6 Surely goodness and mercy shall follow me all the days of my life: and I will dwell in the house of the LORD forever .

Just like sheep, we sometimes need the quite time the good shepherd gives us in Bible study and prayer time.

Chronic stress often causes the body to store fat due to increased cortisol levels which have been released in the stress response. Don't get the wrong idea though, normal cortisol levels are useful to the body. Cortisol increases amino acids, converts amino acids to glucose for use as energy, counteracts inflammation and allergies, helps maintain blood volume and blood pressure, resists stress to the body, and maintains mood and emotional stability.

But once we get too much cortisol we start to see a diminishing of cellular utilization of glucose, increased blood sugar levels, decreased protein synthesis, increased protein breakdown, which leads to muscle breakdown, and demineralization of bone, which can lead to osteoporosis. Excess cortisol interferes with skin regeneration and healing, and can lead to increased allergies, infections, and degenerative disease.

The next time you see someone who looks ten years older than they really are, stress could be the reason why.

Rest

Rest is essential to good health. God has even given us the principle of taking one day each week off from work, which we as Christians now take on Sunday.

Exodus 23:12
Six days thou shalt do thy work, and on the seventh day thou shalt rest: that thine ox and thine ass may rest , and the son of thy handmaid, and the stranger, may be refreshed.

Exodus 33:14
And he said, My presence shall go with thee, and I will give thee rest .

Matthew 11:28
Come unto me, all ye that labour and are heavy laden, and I will give you rest.

Matthew 11:29
Take my yoke upon you, and learn of me; for I am meek and lowly in heart: and ye shall find rest unto your souls.

Of course, the Bible speaks not only of physical rest, but of spiritual rest. However; peace inside from God equals a good night's rest for your physical well-being as well.

Matthew 26:45
Then cometh he to his disciples, and saith unto them, Sleep on now, and take your rest: behold, the hour is at hand, and the Son of man is betrayed into the hands of sinners.

Even beyond the one day a week to rest, we need to get a good night's sleep every night. The body just can't function without adequate rest to recover.

One recent report showed that people who are deprived of sleep eat close to 300 calories more a day than they do when they are well-rested. This probably explains why other research shows that those who do not sleep more than five and half hours a night gain belly fat.

Lack of sleep has been found to lower levels of leptin in the body, a hormone that helps signal the body it is full. Other problems associated with lack of sleep include constipation, stomach ulcers, depression, and heart disease.

Not only is it bad for our health not to get enough rest, just preventing accidents alone is a good enough reason to get a good night's sleep. The U.S. Department of Transportation reports that lack of sleep is responsible for 1,550 deaths and 40,000 injuries each year.

What is a good amount of time to sleep? There are disagreements about what is appropriate, but most opinions wind up around 8 hours a night.

But how do you get a good night's rest if you can't fall asleep at night? A lot of folks these days can't sleep because of all the sugar they eat. Just one more reason to stay clear of sugar is its effects on a good night's sleep. The inflammation alone sugar causes can keep you awake with aches and pains. Please, if you can't rest at night, try changing your diet to healthier food before turning to sleeping pills that may be addictive and have other side effects.

One supplement I might suggest for a good night's rest would be ZMA. Taken about 30 minutes before bed time, it really helps me sleep soundly. ZMA consists of zinc, magnesium, and vitamin B-6. Also keep it as dark as possible in your room. The bedroom should represent a place of rest in your mind. Do not watch TV in your bedroom. TV viewing stimulates the mind, meaning it takes longer to fall asleep. It adds more light to a room which lowers the amount of melatonin your body produces.

Of course, you may have also heard that too much sleep is bad too. It is, therefore, no surprise that the Bible tells us that too much sleep can, at the very least, lead to poverty.

Proverbs 6:9-11
9 How long wilt thou sleep, O sluggard? when wilt thou arise out of thy sleep? 10 Yet a little sleep, a little slumber, a little folding of the hands to sleep: 11 So shall thy poverty come as one that travelleth, and thy want as an armed man.

Gideon

Take the story of Gideon from the book of Judges chapters 6 and 7. God used a test to find whom he wanted to go with Gideon into battle. God was going to use Gideon to defeat the Midianites, and God wanted men that had faith and that were careful going into battle. God said, at first, that all men that were afraid to go into battle should go home, but then next God told Gideon in Judges 7:5, "Every one that lappeth of the water with his tongue, as a dog lappeth, him shalt thou set by himself; likewise every one that boweth down upon his knees to drink."

The Bible goes on to say in Judges 7:6-7, "And the number of them that lapped, putting their hand to their mouth, were three hundred men: but all the rest of the people bowed down upon their knees to drink water. And the LORD said unto Gideon, By the three hundred men that lapped will I save you, and deliver the Midianites into thine hand: and let all the other people go every man unto his place."

So, the men that drank carefully from the water in a way that the enemy could not sneak up on were kept on for the battle. God wanted the faithful and the careful chosen for the battle.

So what lesson is that for living a healthy life? You should trust God for your health, but don't expect God to support being careless in your lifestyle choices, eating and drinking whatever you want without thought to the consequences. Be alert pay attention to what is going on with your body. Take responsibility for everything that goes into your body whether it's food, medicine, or supplements. Read the material the pharmacist gives you with your prescriptions. Know what goes into your body. Take nothing for granted.

Worry

Sometimes worry can cause the things we worry about. We all do it, unfortunately. I'm no different. Even as I write this book I have worries in the back of my mind. It's important to remind ourselves that worry doesn't solve any problems, it just creates problems. We bring the problems of tomorrow onto ourselves today, and then we cause ourselves health issues worrying about things that may or may not happen.

Here are some verses from the Bible concerning worry:

Philippians 4:6-7
6 Be careful for nothing; but in every thing by prayer and supplication with thanksgiving let your requests be made known unto God. 7 And the peace of God, which passeth all understanding, shall keep your hearts and minds through Christ Jesus.

Be careful for nothing basically means be anxious for nothing. Don't worry.

Luke 12:22-26
22 And he said unto his disciples, Therefore I say unto you, Take no thought for your life, what ye shall eat; neither for the body, what ye shall put on. 23 The life is more than meat, and the body is more than raiment. 24 Consider the ravens: for they neither sow nor reap; which neither have storehouse nor barn; and God feedeth them: how much more are ye better than the fowls? 25 And which of you with taking thought can add to his stature one cubit? 26 If ye then be not able to do that thing which is least, why take ye thought for the rest?

Jesus isn't saying don't plan for the future here, but simply not to worry about the future.

Matthew 6:34
34 Take therefore no thought for the morrow: for the morrow shall take thought for the things of itself. Sufficient unto the day is the evil thereof.

I believe Jesus is saying don't bring the problems of tomorrow here today.

Philippians 4:19
19 But my God shall supply all your need according to his riches in glory by Christ Jesus.

Biblically, we can plan for the future and pray about things that concern us, but worrying and agonizing over what may come just takes all the joy out of today, and solves nothing.

We all know that stressing too much is bad for our bodies, and the biggest cause of stress today is worry. Think about all the things we worry about, most likely health is among them, so how does it make sense to worry about health when worry destroys health in the form of stress on our bodies?

Gluttony

Did you know overeating is a sin? Christians laugh at overeating sometimes, even though it's a sin just as much as drinking and smoking.

Don't get me wrong it's good to laugh and not take life too seriously, but I think sometimes the reality of what eating junk food does to a person sometimes escapes us. The idea that overeating or that gluttony is a sin is something we just sort of sweep under the rug and ignore.

Dwight L. Moody, evangelist and founder of the Moody Bible Institute, once said he was asked to pray for a preacher friend of his that was sick, but he refused saying he would not do it because the preacher ate everything in sight. Moody said, "Why should I pray for God to cancel out what he's done to his body 'til he repents."

Now I'm not saying I believe we shouldn't pray for somebody who gets sick. I only mention Moody's position to illustrate a point. We have to take responsibility for what we do to our bodies. We can't eat processed junk food poison and sit all day long without expecting to see some form of negative consequence to our body. Junk food leads to gluttony simply because the more sugar we eat, the more our bodies crave in order to get the same level of satisfaction the next time we eat. Sugar is like an addictive drug.

Deuteronomy puts the drunkard, rebel, and the glutton in the same context.

Deuteronomy 21:20
And they shall say unto the elders of his city, This our son is stubborn and rebellious, he will not obey our voice; he is a glutton, and a drunkard.

And, further on in Proverbs 23, the drunkard and glutton are put in the same context.

Proverbs 23:21
For the drunkard and the glutton shall come to poverty: and drowsiness shall clothe a man with rags.

Proverbs 28:7
Whoso keepeth the law is a wise son: but he that is a companion of riotous men shameth his father.

Apparently, riotous men can be translated into the word "gluttons" if you compare to the New American Standard version which changes "companion of riotous men," shown in the King James Version, to "companion of gluttons".

When you also consider how many times fasting is mentioned in the Bible, you have to come to the conclusion that food is something that may be enjoyed, but shouldn't control us. Self-control and putting God before everything else, including food, is something I think it's safe to say the Bible teaches us.

The next couple of verses illustrate how the Bible depicts someone negatively that makes their belly God in their life.

Philippians 3:18-19
18 (For many walk, of whom I have told you often, and now tell you even weeping, that they are the enemies of the cross of Christ: 19 Whose end is destruction, whose God is their belly, and whose glory is in their shame, who mind earthly things.

This next verse has been used for years by preachers illustrating why we shouldn't smoke, but, if it can be used for smoking, then it seems logical that it could also be used to warn us not to put harmful foods into our bodies as well.

1 Corinthians 6:19-20
What? know ye not that your body is the temple of the Holy Ghost which is in you, which ye have of God, and ye are not your own? 20 For ye are bought with a price: therefore glorify God in your body, and in your spirit, which are God's.

The craving for food got the children of Israel in trouble:

Psalm 78:17-24
17 And they sinned yet more against him by provoking the most High in the wilderness. 18 And they tempted God in their heart by asking **meat for their lust**. 19 Yea, they spake against God; they said, Can God furnish a table in the wilderness? 20 Behold, he smote the rock, that the waters gushed out , and the streams overflowed; can he give bread also? can he provide flesh for his people? 21 Therefore the

LORD heard this, and was wroth: so a fire was kindled against Jacob, and anger also came up against Israel; 22 Because they believed not in God, and trusted not in his salvation: 23 Though he had commanded the clouds from above, and opened the doors of heaven, 24 And had rained down manna upon them to eat, and had given them of the corn of heaven.

Again, this is just another example showing that the Bible teaches us that we can be guilty of putting our food cravings above God.

Now we have to assume that God would not have us to hurt ourselves on purpose. So, doesn't it proceed logically that we are going against the will of God when we put food to our mouths that we know is not healthy or when we put too much food to our mouth making it harmful to our bodies?

Obviously, God wants us to enjoy life. He gave us everything in nature, including sunshine that provides vitamin D, and good tasty natural food that is healthy for us if we'd just eat it. I think if you monitor your weight on a regular basis you can tell really quickly whether or not you are relying on food a little too much in your life.

Eat in moderation. God gives us good sweet stuff like honey to eat, but warns us against over indulging with it.

Proverbs 25:16
16 Hast thou found honey? eat so much as is sufficient for thee, lest thou be filled therewith, and vomit it.

1 Corinthians 10:31
31 Whether therefore ye eat , or drink , or whatsoever ye do , do all to the glory of God.

Be Fit for Your Spouse

People tend to get complacent about fitness after marriage when really we should be more motivated to work out and eat right than ever because we have the added incentive of having someone who would, more than likely, appreciate our efforts. Isn't it funny that we tend to diet and exercise more when we are dating than when have someone who has promised to be with us until death do us part?

The Bible teaches us that we should put others first. Jesus put others above himself. Husbands and wives are told to love one another. Getting in shape for your spouse is a great gift for them and for yourself. By being a good example, you will help motivate your spouse to live a healthy lifestyle as well.

There is sometimes a big gulf between husbands and wives in the area of appearance. Men are created with the tendency to focus on how a woman looks, while women tend to focus more on emotional issues like feeling secure. Therefore, women tend to get upset and feel insecure if their husbands don't appreciate their looks. Living a healthy lifestyle can put some balance on this issue. Both husband and wife can look better for each other by simply eating healthier and being more active, thereby bringing a greater level of confidence to each spouse. Thus, the end result is more happiness, affection, and security in the marriage. Junk food can also mess with a person's emotions causing depression and anxiety, which isn't a good combination for healthy communication in a marriage.

A husband is commanded to love his wife as Christ loved the church. Jesus loved us and gave Himself for us, even though we didn't deserve it. So, for his part, the husband is held accountable for his attitude toward his wife. From the wife's standpoint, she should want to be as lovely, both outwardly and inwardly, for her husband, just as we all should want to live a life that's pleasing to God.

Men especially can make a huge difference in their spouse's health by simply leading by example. Jesus showed a humble leadership by washing His disciple's feet. He lived a perfect life as an example to us all. The spouse that does the grocery shopping has the power to fill the cabinets with healthy alternatives to sugary junk food.

The Bible says, that a man should love his wife like his own body.

Ephesians 5:28
28 So ought men to love their wives as their own bodies. He that loveth his wife loveth himself.

Now, as a test of logic, how much can you love your wife if you don't love your own body enough to take care of it?

I'm not saying, of course, that the physical outweighs the spiritual Biblically, but what I am saying is that God never meant for us to completely ignore the physical. God created everything after all. He is the one that ordained marriage and created the rules we should follow in marriage. For instance, no man can live for long without eating. No matter how spiritual he is, he has to feed the physical body at some point or he will die. So, we have to conclude that for everything there needs to be a balance in life.

Living a healthy lifestyle is a win, win, both spiritually and physically. Not only does a person have a much better chance of living a longer more productive life, but you stand a much better chance at having a happy married life too.

It's easy for us to rationalize almost anything. I really believe that most Christians have talked themselves into believing there isn't anything wrong with eating junk food, and, in fact, they probably believe that by totally ignoring the condition of their physical body, somehow that makes them more spiritual. Nothing could be further from the truth, unless you are sacrificing your health while doing some service for the Lord, there is no reason to believe that God would ever have anybody ignore their physical well-being.

A happy marriage also lends itself to making a couple even healthier beyond what they get from the exercise and healthy foods they consume. Happiness and joy are essential to good health. Having a depressed, negative attitude can be as dangerous as smoking a pack of cigarettes every day. So, it's wise to take our physical well-being seriously for ourselves, our spouses, and to be good examples to our entire families. The Bible says, we reap what we sew. I think that includes taking care of our physical bodies as well as our spiritual needs.

Mental and Spiritual Health

Our spiritual well-being has a direct effect on our mental well-being which, in turn, has a direct effect on our physical well-being. Ignoring the spiritual influences on one's life can have undesirable effects on our physical health.

The mind and the body go hand in hand. Issues already discussed in this book, like avoiding worry and being slow to anger, all stem from the heart and the mind and can eventually cause negative consequences in the body. For example, a new study finds that a person suffering from feelings and thoughts of loneliness is more likely to die earlier than someone who doesn't feel alone.

Another lesson from the Bible from Proverbs 23:7 states, "For as he thinketh in his heart, so is he". Our thoughts control who we are and what we become.

If one thinks of oneself inside as being overweight, non-athletic, and out of shape, that person may never attempt to overcome their physical limitations by exercising and eating healthy. That is, if they feel like it's hopeless because of the negative mental picture they have of themselves, that's likely the actual picture everyone else will see as well. If, on the other hand, someone sees themselves as someone that is athletic, determined, or just has a positive healthy image of themselves in general, they are more likely to make sure that the outside matches the mental image they have of themselves on the inside.

First it's the thought. Then the body goes into action. World famous body builders like Arnold Schwarzenegger often speak of visualizing where they want to be before working out. They focus their minds on the muscle while they are training it, and they imagine what they want their body to look like before they begin each workout session.

Being Wisely Cautious

Proverbs 22:3
A prudent man foreseeth the evil, and hideth himself: but the simple pass on, and are punished.

Some may conclude that eating organic foods and staying away from genetically modified produce and meat with antibiotics and hormones is being a bit overly cautious; however, as the Bible points out, the wise man sees danger coming and tries to avoid it, while the simple go forward without taking thought of the future and suffer for it. We really can't be certain what consequences may be caused by eating GMO's and meat containing antibiotics and hormones. We can only speculate. But anytime poison is put into food, as in the case of some genetically modified foods for the purpose of insect control, it's time to be think twice about eating it. If it kills bugs, what might it be doing to our bodies?

Take the practice of antibiotics being given to our livestock. Some doctors and scientists are saying that the use of antibiotics for livestock is creating new antibiotic-resistant bacteria forms of staph. We know that people who are given excessive amounts of antibiotics over time can create resistant strains of viruses and bacteria that antibiotics can't cure in the future. Consequently now scientists are telling us to hold off on taking antibiotics until it's necessary. So it just makes sense that we shouldn't be eating antibiotics in our food supply every day.

It seems that more and more I hear of people requiring surgery because of infections that antibiotics can't cure. It is something to be aware of and maybe just a little scared of.

I also wonder what effect all those antibiotics have on the good bacteria we have in our guts for digestion, without which good health is nearly impossible. It is known that taking antibiotics in general kills good as well as bad bacteria and we need good bacteria for immune system health. This is one reason why taking probiotics can be a good idea especially if you have had to take antibiotics recently.

Watching one's weight and keeping track of where you are physically in terms of exercise and fitness level is another wise move to avoid illness. Let's face it, we are in a world that is under the penalty of sin. There's a curse on this Earth and we all feel pain and suffering because of it, but a wise person sees ways of avoiding potential pain and suffering for themselves and their families whenever possible. Sometimes all we can do is be a good example for our loved ones in terms of living a healthy lifestyle. Trust me, it does make a difference, even if they don't always take to it as much as you do.

It's so interesting to me that almost every food that God has given us to eat has such great health benefits for us in its basic natural form. If God didn't mean for us to live at a higher level of health than we are living in this country right now, I doubt He would have provided such healthy food for us to eat. America is so blessed right now, but we are more or less squandering that blessing by eating foods that have been altered by man to supposedly taste good and be more convenient, but in reality are nothing more than tasty cigarettes. There really isn't much difference between drinking a six pack of sodas a day and smoking half a pack of cigarettes, especially if you throw in a lifestyle of lying around the house and not exercising.

We are all going to die unless the Lord comes back before then, but why rush it? How is that wise when healthy foods can be just as enjoyable as garbage foods if we just let them? Sure, it takes a little more work to prepare, but the effort is worth it if you can avoid a few surgeries and hospital visits.

Healthy Attitudes

More and more studies are showing that it is what's on the inside that will affect a person's health more than anything else. A person with a sense of humor, or a positive outlook on life is thought to live longer than someone with a negative outlook on life.

One of the reasons, of course, is that, as we all know, stress puts a huge demand on the body. As a result, when your lifetime outlook is down and depressed, it takes its toll on you over the years. Happy people usually – not always – but usually, live longer.

For examples we might consider some of the great comedians of yesteryear like Bob Hope, who always had something humorous to say about almost anything or place he was at in his life. Hope lived to be 100. Even on his deathbed he was joking around. Hope, when asked where he wanted to be buried, told his wife, "Surprise me".

The great comic, Jack Benny, lived to be 80. No one alive today could match Jack Benny's comedic timing.

George Burns, another comedian from the golden age of television lived to be 100. Like Jack Benny toward his wife Mary Livingstone, Burns was famous for the great love he shared with his wife, Gracie Allen. Burns stated that, while he looked forward to being 100 years old, he also looked forward to being with Gracie in heaven. Gracie Allen had died in 1969 at the age of 69. Upon being interred with Gracie, the crypt's marker was changed to, "Gracie Allen & George Burns—Together Again." George had said that he wanted Gracie to have top billing.

At the time of this writing, Larry Torch, who played Corporal Randolph Agarn on *F-Troop*, is still alive and well at age 89. Groucho Marx of the Marx Brothers movies and the game show *You Bet Your Life*, lived to be 86. Frank Cady, who played Sam Drucker on *Green Acres* and *Petticoat Junction*, died recently at the age of 96.

Then there's Mr. Warmth, Don Rickles, who comes across as a mean old man, but you know he must have a really huge sense of humor to tell some of the jokes he does. Even the President is fair game for Rickle's humor when the President is in the same room. Rickles is still currently going strong, insulting everyone at the young age of 86.

Dick Van Dyke of the *Dick Van Dyke Show* is also 86 as of this writing. He may also be a good example of the effects of dancing on longevity considering his footwork on *Mary Poppins* and the end of *Night of the Museum*.

Andy Griffith is another classic TV sitcom star who is also known for his country gospel singing. He passed away in 2012, at a nice old age of 86.

Now compare that to the great health guru, Jack Lalaine, who lived to be 96 years old. Everyone knows that if anyone ever had the perfect diet and exercise plan in life it was Jack Lalaine, but it's very interesting to note how many people known for their sense of humor have lived as long as, or longer than, a man who quite arguably had the most healthy lifestyle of anyone on the planet in the last 100 years.

Proverbs 17:22
A merry heart doeth good like a medicine: but a broken spirit drieth the bones.

My examples admittedly are less than scientific. After all, no one can prove that comedians who live long lives have had great positive attitudes in their personal lives, but it has been proven again and again that stress causes us to age faster. Eating right, exercising, and keeping a good healthy outlook on life are essential to long life. There are those, of course, who break all the rules and still manage to live longer lives than those that do live healthy lives.

Have you ever met someone who takes themselves way too seriously? You can't joke with them. You can't play around with them because, brother, the minute you do, they go off. Then you meet others that always have a smile on their face and love to kid around, almost to the point of nausea. Still, how would you rather feel in life? Be happy or be miserable – in the long, run barring the usual ups and downs in life, it's really our choice. Knowing, as we do, that whatever emotional state we are in has a lot to do with how long we live, isn't it wise to look at our glasses as half full instead of half empty? If you happen to drop that glass, just laugh about it. Your heart will thank you. Seriously, the way we handle stress can be as valuable to our health as a good doctor, not smoking, or eating organic vegetables and grass fed beef – possibly more so.

Some people act as if they are in a constant state of war readiness. Their bodies and faces are always tense. You can just see it on their faces and in their actions. You know the type I'm talking about. Just try to crack a little joke, and you'll get a look from then like you just came off a UFO from Mars.

Having an intense personality can come in handy when doing difficult jobs that take lots of concentration, but individuals of this personality type need to know when to deflate. Just imagine the stress on the heart and the rest of the body when a person is constantly flexed for some major catastrophe.

I speak as one that has had to work on developing ways to manage stress myself. Going for a walk, watching an old black and white comedy on TV, or just exercising in general are some ways I relax. Personally, I have to add, that as much as I love action shows like *24* with super-agent Jack Bauer, watching programs of such high intensity on a daily basis can take a toll on your nerves after a while. It's like putting yourself into a combat situation, which is definitely not good right before bed time. Finding quite time to read the Bible, or other books in general, is a good way to relax.

I definitely would recommend avoiding watching a typical modern day horror movie. Things we watch affect the mind which in turn has an impact on our body . Think about what seeing ruthless murder and torture scenes on a movie screen does to a person's mental health over time. It's no wonder people are so stressed out and overly serious about everything in life. People who have never even been in a war can literally witness gruesome experiences on a giant movie screen that even seasoned combat vets are not likely to see.

Some parents see no problem at all letting their children see some of this stuff, and I can only imagine the anxiety and fear that must trigger in these kids. Things that we see as children can stick in our minds for the rest of our lives. I still remember the fear I had of vampire movies as a child, and those movies were nothing compared to ultra-realistic blood and gore effects featured in movies today.

Negative stress adds up in our bodies and minds. Positive stress like exercise and accomplishing a goal at work can be beneficial to us physically as long as it isn't something that is prolonged. Even exercise has now been found to have a cutoff point at about an hour a day. Running all day marathons for instance has actually been found to scar the heart. A challenging workout that lasts for about an hour a day is what you want to shoot for. Any more highly intensive exercise than that and you start to see diminishing results.

We can't help hitting stressful times in our lives. It's inevitable, and it is also inevitable that the stress may affect us negatively unless we can handle it in a positive way. The one thing you definitely don't want to do is to add unnecessary stress to your daily life. It's good to relax at least once a day and watch something easy on the mind, especially right before bed. Read a book. Personally, I like to watch an old black and white comedy to relax my mind before calling it a day. Laughter is great medicine and the old shows have a calming effect on a person's mind.

Getting a good night's sleep, by the way, has a lot to do with what kind of attitude you have the next day. Being tired makes every problem in the world appear insurmountable. Not to mention how cranky and just plain ornery one can get after not getting a good night's sleep.

Now the biggest way we can have a good, healthy attitude is to focus on our spiritual life. Man is without a doubt a spiritual being. As a Christian, I believe that there is nothing more important to a healthy life than taking care of the spiritual aspects of life first. Having peace inside through trusting Jesus Christ is about the only way I know of to really be able to relax in life. Life is always hammering at us from every side; it's always good to know that through Jesus Christ we have God watching over us as his own children. Without having peace with God, it's impossible to have peace in life.

Even as Christians, we miss out on so much in our health by not following Biblical teachings. Loving one another, not rendering evil for evil, being slow to anger, not worrying, all Biblical principles that if followed can keep a man or woman a lot happier, and, in turn, lead to a much healthier life. We age much faster than we should just because of the stress we create by worry, anger, grudges, and so on that we hold in our hearts.

You notice the Bible doesn't say anywhere not to rest until you have your revenge. It doesn't say to worry because you have no chance of making it. It doesn't say to get mad when someone gets in your way on the road. It says to live peacefully with all men, and that God knows every need we have. Think of all the needless stress we put on ourselves because we just don't turn our worries over to God and let go of negative attitudes and feelings that the Bible plainly calls sin.

It isn't easy but to truly address every area of our health we have to address our spiritual health first. The Bible says in 1 Timothy 4:8:

For bodily exercise profiteth little: but godliness is profitable unto all things, having promise of the life that now is, and of that which is to come.

Notice it doesn't say that there is no profit to exercise, only that it the profit is small. Of course, in terms of all eternity in heaven, everything on Earth that we do for our physical life is of little profit because it is only temporary. Unless the Lord returns first, we will physically die eventually no matter what we do, but godliness shows us profit after we die and while we live as the verse says, **"having promise of the life that now is"**.

So there is double reward for putting the spiritual before the physical. I believe the reward here and now is a good relationship with God, as well as healthier relationships with our family that, in turn, makes us healthier physically.

As I've said before, we run into stress all the time in our lives, sometimes because of problems we create and sometimes it's things we have no control over, but why add to our grief by adding worry, anger, and spite to the mix?

Proverbs 15:1 gives us a great way to avoid stress in our lives:

1 A soft answer turneth away wrath: but grievous words stir up anger.

Avoid anger and you can avoid a lot of stress. Getting along with your fellow man, or at least not holding anything against your fellow man, can go a long way toward living stress free. I mean, let's face it, there are some people out there that no matter how nice you are to them they will never return the favor, but that only hurts them on the inside. Returning evil for evil only escalates things, and before I go any further I'm not referring to physical self-defense here, but to going out of one's way to pay someone back for the purpose of revenge.

Talk about unhealthy, the story of the Hatfields and the McCoys is a classic example of why people should read their Bibles a little more carefully. It's a classic true life story of two families seeking revenge on the other killing each other off for a senseless family feud.

They could have spared themselves a whole lot of trouble if they would have just read 1 Thessalonians 5:15:

15 See that none render evil for evil unto any man; but ever follow that which is good, both among yourselves, and to all men.

And Matthew 5:39:

39 But I say unto you, That ye resist not evil: but whosoever shall smite thee on thy right cheek, turn to him the other also.

These days we might not necessarily shoot it out with our neighbors, but seeking to harm others through other methods for the purpose of revenge only hurts everyone involved. The moral to the story is that we should live peaceably with all men, for their sakes and for your own health. You don't have to get shot to have anger and bitterness eat you up on the inside.

Another thing you might keep in mind in having a healthy mindset and reduced stress level – don't watch the news 24 hours a day. Seriously, I can't think of anything more nerve-racking than what's on the news. And don't forget, news anchors make money by worrying you. Fox News may claim to be fair and balanced, but it definitely isn't balanced on the stress meter. None of the news stations or programs are. Unfortunately, few people stop what they are doing to watch broadcasts about good news, so the more cataclysmic and depressing the news is, the more it gets run over and over again. This, in turn, gives the viewer a very discouraging outlook about the current situation in the world. Sure, everything they say may be true, but how many good things could the news also report about if they thought anybody would watch?

Just look at some of these news headlines I pulled up on the internet within the same hour of this writing.

Crackdown on painkiller abuse fuels new wave of heroin addiction

US blamed for on-going massacre in Syria

Unemployment in Greece hits 22%

and my favorite news item this hour,

This Is the Way the World Ends? Volcanoes Could Darken World

Yeah, the news is bad, and even though we can't really do anything to change it, per se, from the safety of our sofas, the inner feelings of stress and hopelessness pile up after a while.

I'm not saying you should keep yourself in the dark, but once the news goes into the repeat cycle, turn the channel or turn it off.

We are all guilty of worry. We all struggle with it at times, and it can cause a lot of harm to the body over time, especially if you add in overeating that comes about when people look for outward solutions.

Jesus warned us not to worry and told us our heavenly Father was looking out for us.

> Matthew 6:25-33
> 25 Therefore I say unto you, Take no thought for your life, what ye shall eat, or what ye shall drink; nor yet for your body, what ye shall put on. Is not the life more than meat, and the body than raiment? 26 Behold the fowls of the air: for they sow not, neither do they reap, nor gather into barns; yet your heavenly Father feedeth them. Are ye not much better than they? 27 Which of you by taking thought can add one cubit unto his stature? 28 And why take ye thought for raiment? Consider the lilies of the field, how they grow; they toil not, neither do they spin: 29 And yet I say unto you, That even Solomon in all his glory was not arrayed like one of these. 30 Wherefore, if God so clothe the grass of the field, which today is, and tomorrow is cast into the oven, shall he not much more clothe you, O ye of little faith? 31 Therefore take no thought, saying, What shall we eat? or, What shall we drink? or, Wherewithal shall we be clothed? 32 (For after all these things do the Gentiles seek:) for your heavenly Father knoweth that ye have need of all these things. 33 But seek ye first the kingdom of God, and his righteousness; and all these things shall be added unto you.

It's not always easy, but if we can learn to trust God with our problems and worries we could see a lot fewer heart attacks in this country. Worry just brings tomorrow's problems here, today, and doesn't really do anything to solve the problem. One of the toughest things in life is to address problems without letting concern drift over to worry. Planning for the future is something the Bible teaches, but when planning turns to fretting you've gone too far. Once we've taken steps that can be done today to address whatever problems we face it's time to pray and let go. I don't believe God wants us to just let things slide, but clearly from what Jesus said, He doesn't want us to put stress upon ourselves needlessly for all the potential problems we have or can dream up.

4 THE SUGAR ADDICTION

Researchers have shown the neurochemical effects of sugar might actually serve as a gateway drug. We can clearly see that sugar is addictive by simply looking at ourselves and others around us.

You might be surprised to learn that in one study, rats given sugar water showed behavior like that of drug addicts. When the sugar had been taken away from them, the rats had signs of drug withdrawal, such as teeth-chattering and the shakes.

Sugar and the taste of sweets stimulate the brain by activating beta endorphin receptor sites according to one study. These are the same chemicals activated by heroin and morphine. But, again, we don't really need a lot of research scientists to tell us that sugar is addictive. All we have to do is look around us.

Just take a trip to your local grocery store. You'll see an alarming number of folks very close to, or over the line of obesity. Obesity rate for adults has doubled what it was thirty years ago. The number of obese children has tripled in the same time period.

If you find yourself obese, or even just a little overweight, I think that just realizing that, not only is sugar fattening, but it is also an addiction, can help put you in the right mindset to overcome your problem, eat right and see amazing results. I think the biggest problem is that people don't see anything wrong with eating junk food. I believe there needs to be a stigma on junk food like there is on cigarettes.

Back to your local grocery store. So, let's look around. You'll see people riding around in power chairs instead of walking. Are they all handicapped? I know there are legitimately disabled individuals riding the power chairs, but, you know, my gut tells me that a lot of people riding power chairs may be just overweight and can't stand the strain of walking around the store, or simply lack the motivation.

One of the pitfalls of over consumption of sugar and lack of exercise is an ever decreasing lack of motivation to get up and be active. This only compounds the ill effects of being overweight. Exercise and activity are key ingredients in a healthy lifestyle. This lack of motivation turns into depression which creates an almost unbearable feeling of helplessness and hopelessness. You can see it in the eyes of most Americans these days. Sugar, like cocaine or methamphetamine, robs individuals of their will to live. Most will blame it on their busy lifestyles. They're tired from a hard day. And, while busy schedules are another stressor that these modern days place on our lives that can hurt our health over time, it doesn't compare with the ill effects of the overconsumption of sugar.

The truth is, the harder your day is, the more energy you need. You won't find lasting energy in a soft drink. Just a momentary pick-me-up from the caffeine, which you can just as easily get in a cup of tea, or a cup of coffee. If you feel drained every day, you need nutrients, not nutrient robbers in your diet. If you can manage to do even 30 minutes of exercise a day you'll reap many benefits over time. One of which will be much greater amounts of sustained energy. The more tired you are, the less you do, the more tired you become and the more sugar you crave. It's another endless cycle.

Research indicates that lack of sleep can cause people to crave more calories. I'll give you one guess what that means to most Americans – more sugar.

You can see how this all adds up. We literally have the walking dead among us. So, if you always feel tired and run down, don't necessarily blame your work schedule. You may want to look at your diet. Some things we can't control. We can't control having to work additional hours, or how many family emergencies happen in a week, but you can control what fuel you put into your body.

Would you put sugar into your gas tank? I take that back. We even do that these days in the form of fermented sugar, known as ethanol, which, by the way, has been known to clump up in sugary lumps in lawn mower gas tanks, causing the gas mixture to be unable to get to the engine.

At any rate, for the sake of an example, would you put a soft drink into your gas tank? That would be fun to see what happens, wouldn't it? No, you want to put the best gas you can into your car. You want it to run smoothly so you don't get stuck on the side of the road or have to pay for costly repairs. The same goes for your body. Why put bad fuel in there and expect your body to run right? It's not going to.

One of the main reasons I think so many people are depressed these days is that they're so out of shape. You can't tell me that having a lower self-image doesn't affect a person in a negative way. On top of that constant pain, being unable to move is not something we normally aspire to in life.

It's not my intention to make anyone feel bad, but people have to admit they have a problem before the problem can be solved. It's not just a matter of vanity as some would have us believe. It's become a matter of life and death. Even the quality of life we have from day to day is suffering thanks to America's eating habits. Sugar causes painful inflammation. That means that as we get older, those normal aches and pains are doubled or tripled. Are the cookies and ice cream worth all that pain? Then there's the weight that makes a person less mobile, which means less exercise and reduces their body's ability to burn calories. It's a never-ending cycle of pain and weight gain, which leads to more pain and more weight gain, as exercise is essential to a healthy life.

How many people back in their younger days said to themselves when I grow up I want to be a 100 pounds overweight and hurt all the time so I can eat my cookies and ice cream? Of course, these days even teens, with all their peer pressure to look good, are seeking the sugar god above looking trim and fit. It's an addiction, there's no doubt about it. When you trade your appearance, your health, your mobility, and the length of days on this earth for anything, it most certainly is an addiction.

As a Christian I believe nothing is supposed to take the place of God in our lives. But clearly, sugar has become a god to many Americans, both Christians and non-believers alike. They just don't seem to realize it.

When I was first getting off of sugar and junk food, I could tell how much more I ached on days I had too much sugar than other days that I ate less sugar. Of course, now sugar is almost non-existent in my diet. I've learned there is a price for sugar, and I'm not willing to pay it. Seriously, is it worth physical pain, inflammation, and extra fat? I don't need or want diabetes or future heart problems.

Bedridden Obese – The Ultimate Victims of Sugar Addiction

The ultimate end of a sugar laden diet is to be bedridden and obese. That is, if you live long enough to get to that point. As further proof that sugar is addictive, we can examine the lives of the bedridden obese, who insanely continue to eat sugary snacks and high fat processed foods even after losing the ability to move from their beds. What has shocked me are those that continue to feed their obese loved ones enough junk food to keep them bedridden. It's like buying alcohol for an alcoholic or drugs for a drug addict. Do they think their loved one is better off as long as they get what they want? How do people justify this madness? Maybe it's just that we as a society believe we are entitled to have everything we want, even though, obviously, sometimes we are not better off with what we want.

Sometimes we just have to say no. Self-reliance has made America great, but now we see Americans freely trading in their self-reliance for the god of sugar. If you have a loved one bedridden from obesity, it's time for some tough love. If you are the only one bringing them food, you have the power to make a change in their life. First, you should work with their doctor to develop a good diet to wean them off of the excess sugar and carbs slowly. If you continue to feed them cakes, ice cream, and cokes while they are bedridden from obesity, you are basically killing your loved one slowly.

Here is a very sad story that happened in America in 2009, to a man who was only 33 years of age. The 550 pound man came home from the hospital after hurting his knee and sat down in his single wide trailer. There he stayed, sitting in his recliner for eight months. By this time his weight had increased to 800 pounds and he had to be cut from the chair, to which he had become physically welded, and taken to the hospital, where he later died of a heart attack. The man had slept and even went to the bathroom in his chair. He was covered with sores. A hole had to be cut out of the trailer to get the man out. It was like something out of a horror picture.

There are many sad aspects to this story. First, the man was neither an alcoholic nor a druggie. In fact, he was a former preacher who had faith that God would heal his leg, according to his wife who took care of him during this time. She said that he read his Bible every day, and had hope that God would heal him.

Admittedly, I have to make some assumptions here, but it does appear evident, from the information from the Associated Press, that his wife no doubt fed the man, and we can only guess what she fed him was enough to make him balloon from 550 pounds to 800 pounds. Yes, a leg injury can make a man gain weight due to a lack of activity, but this level of weight gain has to be the result of massive junk food and sugar intake. The woman no doubt loved her husband, but she most likely fed him the wrong kinds of foods, which eventually led to his demise. This kind of story has been happening more and more frequently in the world since obesity has been on the rise.

In the UK, a 980 pound man had to be transported in an ambulance that was special made to handle his size. He admits his problem started by compulsive eating initiated by traumatic events in his life. Specially made wheel chairs had to be made, and the door frame was already widened from a previous trip the hospital. The interesting thing here is, the man can't get up, so you have to wonder who was feeding him. Did he have pizza and soda delivered to his door every day? More likely someone, some well-meaning loved one was feeding him everything he wanted every day. Why, because it might make him sad to have to eat real food? The logic escapes me. We live in a day where we've gotten the idea that it's wrong to say no, as if not getting sugary treats was worse than death itself.

These stories are classic examples of what happens when over indulging in sugar causes insulin insensitivity. The person's body no longer pays attention to the insulin and can no longer ever feel satisfied. That's the risk you take when drink those sodas every day.

Are You a Slave to Food?

Are you a slave to food? Does your food add to your energy and feed your muscle, or does it add to your body's fat storage units located in your stomach, hips, and thighs? Food can be a powerful servant that keeps us going, and even keeps us alive, but it can also be a cruel master that some would rather bow before at the expense of not only their outward appearance, but their health as well.

Take the recent case of the teenager living in the UK who had to have the walls of her home cut out in order to get her to the hospital. It took a team of 40 people to get her out and on her way to the hospital. She had complaints of diabetes, kidney disease, spinal problems and respiratory failure, all at the age of 19. Her choice of food included processed ready-meals, sandwiches, packs of peanuts, crisps, sausages, pasties, chips, chocolate and chunks of cheese with bottles of coke or pints of milk. The girl was quoted as saying that food was an addiction to her like drugs or alcohol. In 2008, the teen, told reporters: "Some people choose heroin, but I've chosen food and it's killing me".

Doctors are now convinced that sugary processed foods have addictive qualities, much like heroin. It's clearly evidenced in cases like that of the 19 year old food addict, but she's not the only one. There are varying degrees of addiction across the world today. More and more people are accepting their bodies with too much fat as if it were normal. Many people may even think that they have a medical issue when, in fact, what they really have is just an eating issue.

Some have just given up and have started campaigns to accept overweight people as they are. Of course, nobody has a right to judge another person based on his or her outward, physical appearance, but I'm convinced that we should judge ourselves in every area of life. How else can a person be wise and see the dangers of their actions before it's too late, whether the danger is physical or spiritual.

Proverbs 22:3
A prudent man foreseeth the evil, and hideth himself: but the simple pass on, and are punished.

I don't believe in labeling someone as fat and then making that person feel unworthy in any way, but at the same time I think making general statements that being overweight is unhealthy is something that needs to be stated and not held in for fear of being politically incorrect. As I've stated before, being overweight is not a sin, but eating more than what is healthy for our bodies is. It's called gluttony.

We live in a society today where personal responsibility gets pushed farther and farther away. Individuals want to make excuses and to blame society, corporations, politicians, and all the rest for their own woes. The unfortunate reality is that, in most cases, we only have ourselves to blame. There are many things we can do to change things for the better. For instance, if we stop buying unhealthy junk food, then the corporations will be forced to sell healthier products.

Recently, the mayor of New York was seeking to outlaw large soft drinks from being sold in town. That isn't really what our founders would have wanted for the government to get involved in. It's not the government's responsibility to enforce healthy living on its populace. It's the responsibility of the individual to take care of themselves. The government's role should be more to the point of requiring accurate labels of the contents in food, including GMO's, not getting involved in limiting what people can or cannot buy in regards to sizes of food and drink products.

It has to be an individual's choice to live healthy. It cannot be forced. A person has to realize that they have a problem with food before they will ever change. Society does need to be more upfront about the addictive nature of junk food and recognize that it is a problem instead of letting people with eating disorders claim their overweight stature is part of who they are. Nobody is born with a soda in their hands, not that we can't be compassionate towards those that suffer from a food addiction, but we need to be honest about it. The first step in overcoming addiction is realizing you have one.

One issue with the outlook of the obesity epidemic in our world right now is that, over time, the idea of what is healthy may become distorted. The more people we know that are overweight, the more we start to think that what might have been considered overweight twenty years ago is now normal. The effects of the weight on our health will not change, but the perception that people have may change with time as people become bigger and bigger.

Master food instead of being its slave. Don't allow junk food into your home, and don't allow food to be taken into a child's room unless you want them to wind up stuck on the bed unable to get up the rest of their life.

The nice thing about healthy food is that tastes good. It fulfills your nutrition needs, and it's not addictive. When was the last time you heard that someone had become obese eating celery, spinach, broccoli, apples, lean meat and drinking unsweetened tea? It doesn't happen, and not just because those foods have fewer calories. It's because they are natural foods, and natural foods aren't addictive. Well I should say you don't hear any morbidly obese tales from people eating health food, though I have heard stories of people becoming overweight or hurting their liver from eating too many oranges. Fruits are not addictive like junk food, but it is possible to eat too much fruit due to the fructose in them. Still, fruit is a much better choice to eat than junk food any day of the week. Just set a limit of one a day per type of fruit. Don't eat 40 oranges a day and not expect some kind of consequences.

Buy food that God made, and avoid foods that man has manipulated or added chemicals to. The more natural the food is the healthier the food choice it is.

Don't add sugar to food, and try to avoid foods in cans that have added chemicals and sugar. Take charge of your life and be free.

I think one of the biggest issues people face today with food is that it becomes God in their life. They lean on it in troubled times. They believe food relieves their stress. The problem with food is it only satisfies temporarily, sometimes not even then for the obese who have to keep eating more and more to find that satisfaction they desperately crave.

If you know somebody that has an eating problem, and everybody reading this probably does, be kind and encourage that person to get outside and find other things to do besides eating for enjoyment in life.

It's sad, but if we are honest about it, even Christians today put food on a pedestal. It's as if it's the last thing they can enjoy without feeling guilty, not realizing that anything that is put above God becomes their god. Perhaps this is why the Bible promotes times of fasting for us to deny food and put God first.

I know it might sound harsh, and I certainly do not want to tell people that eating ice cream in moderation is a terrible sin, but I think at some point we have to weigh the consequences of eating that ice cream. If it starts to noticeably alter our health in a negative fashion, then maybe we need to step back and ask ourselves, "Just how important is junk food?"

It's interesting that God created so many sweet things to eat like apples and berries, but He never created a cake and ice cream tree. Again, eating ice cream isn't necessarily a sin in and of itself, but I certainly think it can be.

Recently, we got a coupon for a free pint of ice cream, and I treated myself to some, which I think is ok to do once in a while. I gained a pound the next day, but I can't prove it was the ice cream. It was my day off from eating healthy, and I have to disclose that I also had some chicken strips from Chick-fil-A that day as well. Imagine though, how much weight you can gain in a year from eating like that if you gained a pound every day. I know there are limits, but we see more and more people that look like they've gained more than a pound a day in a year.

Food should be one of our tools to use to better our health. It should be enjoyable, but if it has become your master, then that sort of takes the enjoyment out of it really.

Healthy fruits and vegetables can be a joy to eat, and you can even enjoy them while losing weight at the same time. The bottom line is the body needs nutrition. That's what God made food for, to provide the necessary nutrients our bodies need to carry out our daily tasks. It's an added bonus that food tastes good. So maybe, just maybe, we all should be a little less greedy and just be happy with natural healthy foods and keep the junk food for the occasional cheat meal.

The best way to beat food addiction, by far, is to systematically replace each bad food choice with a healthy choice until all that's left is healthy food. Start with sodas. Replace them with water or tea, no fruit juices. Eventually processed sugary foods will be a thing of the past and the fat will come off naturally one day at a time. You will be amazed by how much your food cravings diminish once you remove added sugars from your diet.

Start an exercise program that fits your physical fitness level. Nothing motivates a person more to eat healthy food than when they realize it's helping them accomplish other goals in life. Goals of physical fitness, of course, rely heavily on what we eat and don't eat.

Make sure you eat before you go to the grocery store, or you'll be more likely to purchase foods based on your cravings than based on good common sense. When shopping, buy frozen fruits instead of canned fruits as they don't usually have as many chemicals added and keep all their nutrients. Plus they don't have sugary syrup added to the mix. Fruit tastes sweet enough as it is, you really don't need syrup added to the amount of sugar you get in fruit.

Take charge of food and be its master not the other way around. Make food work for you by doing what it was intended to by God, and that's give you energy and nutrients not make you sick and fat.

What Sugar Does to Your Body

There are many problems and concerns associated with, or thought to be associated with, the intake of sugar specifically fructose, which is the unhealthy portion of sugar. Fructose, which makes up almost half or more of refined sugar, causes your brain to believe you're starving even when you are full.

Sugar damages collagen and elastin in our skin, turning them dry and brittle, which then produces wrinkles. How ironic that if we eat like a kid with cokes, ice cream, candy, etc., we'll look old faster, but if we eat like an older, wiser person would in theory, we'll look younger, more like a kid.

Excessive fructose consumption is believed to contribute to the development of non-alcoholic fatty liver disease.

Insulin resistance may affect the hippocampus, a part of the brain critical for learning and remembering facts and events. Insulin resistance is a consequence of excess fructose consumption.

Pancreatic tumor cells use fructose to divide and proliferate, or multiply.

Too much sugar causes diabetes, heart disease and stroke, according to the American Heart Association.

Fruit juice contains more fructose than simply eating a piece of fruit, and studies show these sugary drinks cause weight gain.

Sugar can hurt your immune system making you more susceptible to colds and flu.

High Fructose Corn Syrup (HFCS) consumption may lead to nonalcoholic fatty liver disease, followed by hepatic insulin resistance and then type 2 diabetes.

Refined sugar contains no fiber, no vitamins, no minerals, no proteins, no fats, no enzymes, only empty calories. Your body has to use nutrients already in your body to process it. So basically sugar robs your body of nutrients.

Unbound fructose, found in large quantities in HFCS, can interfere with your heart's use of minerals such as magnesium, copper and chromium. Fructose in fruit comes with the nutrients necessary for your body to process the fructose. So you can see how processed foods and sodas could turn dangerous over a short period of time.

Sugar increases instances of tooth decay. Sugar makes the blood very thick and sticky, inhibiting much of the blood flow into the minute capillaries that supply our gums and teeth with vital nutrients. So, we wind up with diseased gums and starving teeth.

Sugar may increase chances of getting gallstones.

Sugar may cause our cells to be robbed of B vitamin, which destroys the cells, and insulin production is inhibited. Low insulin production means a high sugar (glucose) level in the bloodstream, which can lead to a confused mental state or unsound mind, and has also been linked with juvenile criminal behavior. TV health guru, Jack Lalanne, claimed that ending his junk food diet as a young teenager saved him from behavioral problems. He suffered from headaches and bulimia, and temporarily dropped out of school at age 14. He reported that before he became health conscious, he had violent episodes, which he attributed to sugar and junk food.

Uneven sugar levels in your blood often cause mood changes, sudden tiredness, constant headache and the desire to eat even more sugar.

Obesity is a major problem in the world today. It's without a doubt caused by diets loaded with sugar, and the fact that we sit more than ever before. Still, even allowing for the sitting all day every day, the tremendous amounts of weight on some unfortunate people these days can only be accounted for in their diets. People are getting bigger than what was once thought physically possible. The problem with a high sugar diet is it never satisfies, and it only makes you want more and more like a very dangerous drug.

If you love yourself and your family it's time to get serious about this dangerous food we are all playing around with. If you have kids it may seem almost impossible to enforce healthy eating habits. With the exception of the occasional treat, having a no tolerance policy for junk food in the home is a great start. After all if it's not there they can't eat it. Of course, then you have to worry what they eat at school, or at their friends' or grandparents' houses.

Obesity rates in boys are especially climbing, going up from 14 percent in 1999-2000, to 18.6 percent in 2009-2010. It's time to put some restrictions on video game and computer time and get those kids outside playing again. I think it's a shame that many schools have gotten rid of recess time. This time is especially important for boys to engage each other in some type of game to get them competitive and motivated and moving. Boys need competition. These days, both boys and girls alike are increasingly becoming living vegetables. It's beyond sad, and if we don't take steps to change it, we are going to have a whole generation that lives more of their lives sick than healthy.

But even so, if kids never got up to play, there wouldn't be half the obesity rate we have now if sugar and junk food weren't added into the mix on top of the lack of physical activity. It's like adding fuel to the fire.

What is the definition of obese? It's anybody that is roughly 30 pounds over their healthy bodyweight.

Recently, USA Today reported that a new government forecast calls for 42% of Americans to end up obese by 2030, and 11% could be severely obese, adding billions of dollars to health care costs. This would mean 32 million more obese people within two decades.

The interesting thing is, it doesn't have to be this way. Almost anybody can lose weight, in most circumstances, by just eating real food and becoming more active. Slow metabolisms are created by unhealthy lifestyle choices, like yo yo dieting. Waiting hours to eat, eating just one meal a day, or living on just crackers one week, which, by the way, isn't healthy, and then going back to eating all the junk food and garbage you ate before the next week only saddles you with a slow metabolism by killing your muscles and causes you gain back all the weight you lost and then some, leaving you weighing more than you did before you started the starvation diet. The preferred method of weight loss is gradual, eating healthy foods that can support your muscles even when you eat fewer calories.

Interestingly enough, the kind of behavior I see in people that causes the most weight gain comes from those that are stuck on the ideas that skipping breakfast, or eating only once or twice a day will result in weight loss. What happened, of course, was they probably saw a drop in their weight at first because they had fewer calories that day. They made the wrong assumption then that this was the way to lose weight. It's a no win situation because the less you eat the slower your metabolism goes. Now you add to that fact that folks with weight issues will then add to their woes by having huge unhealthy dinners and big desserts afterward, and this after they've slowed their metabolism to a crawl.

Occasionally, you can skip a meal here and there and lose a bit, but over a prolonged time period it can backfire on you. You have to keep your metabolism going. You have to remember that the body is created to adapt itself to whatever amount of calories you put into it. Excessive calories go to fat storage. Going hungry may make the body start to use stored fat, but at the same time the body gets a signal to slow down its overall calorie burning to conserve energy. Also you have to remember the body tends to eat muscle when you go hungry. Muscle aids metabolism.

Think of your metabolism as a fire in your stomach. When you want to build a fire and keep it going you don't throw huge logs on top of a tiny fire. That will just snuff it out. No, what you do is start with tiny twigs fed into the fire every little bit until the fire builds bigger, at which time, you can add bigger logs to the fire. Now what if you wait too long before adding another log? The fire goes out. In your body, what would happen is that big log, or piece of chocolate cake is instantly turned into fat.

So, what would make for nice twigs to start the fire of metabolism going? Start with green vegetables, maybe some spinach, or some kind of leafy green vegetable, but hold the sugary dressing. Have an apple, and don't forget the protein, such as a little bit of chicken or fish. Eat small healthy snacks every couple of hours, and let the fire build up. By the end of the day you'll feel fuller, and you won't feel the need to fill your gut like a camel loading up on water heading into the desert. Over time your metabolism will be higher and the occasional piece of cake won't do quite as much damage – and I said **occasional**. A piece of cake a day is a recipe for a big gut, unless you are a world class athlete who can burn all those calories off every day.

Of course, we have to go back to discussing weight training in terms of increasing metabolism. The more muscle you have the higher your rate of metabolism. The simple reason is that muscle eats fat and calories to stay alive. That's why weight training is so important to aiding in fat loss. This is also why women have a harder time keeping off the fat than men do. Sorry ladies! It's just harder for you to keep off weight, which means you should be watching your sugar intake all the more if you want to stay trim.

A lot of women are afraid to lift weights because it might make them look like a guy, or maybe they're afraid they'll look like a female body builder on steroids. First of all, you would have to actually take steroids, and secondly, the amount of time a woman would have to spend in the gym to have bulky, oversized muscles is way more than the average person could do, unless they were earning a living at body building. Women do not have as much testosterone as men, so they can't build muscle as readily as men.

The next thing to keep in mind is that muscle appears thinner than fat. The only place fat looks good is in the face and that's when it's in the right areas, and not under the chin.

So, building muscle will help make you look thinner especially as you get older. The interesting thing about muscle is that it weighs more than fat, but again makes you look thin and athletic in appearance verses round and heavy looking.

5 DON'T DIET, EAT HEALTHY

Most people go wrong in their weight loss strategy because they start out thinking about it all wrong. Most people put all of their faith in a magic diet plan, but the cold hard truth is that short term temporary diets aren't good for anything but short term results that might shave off a few pounds that eventually come right back. Most diet plans will fail you because of their short term nature. A good diet is one you can stick with the rest of your life that focuses first on health then on fat loss as the primary goal.

Focus on eating healthy foods – real foods that aren't processed, in a can or have added chemicals and sugar. I can almost guarantee that anybody who replaces processed foods with real food will see not only weight loss, but muscle gain with strength training, and overall better health. When I say real food, I mean fruits, vegetables, and lean meat that you have to cook yourself, preferably with no hormones or antibiotics. Chances are, if it's already cooked and in a can, or wrapped in plastic, it's not any good for you. There are degrees of course. If you have to eat something processed, then you should at least pay close attention to the nutrition label, particularly the amount of sugar, and the list of ingredients inside. For the best results, however, you should primarily ditch processed foods and take the time to prepare your own meals.

It really is that simple. Real food satisfies your body with the nutrients it needs, and your body eventually gets the message and stops constantly hungering for more. You'll always be hungry eating junk because your body never gets the nutrients it needs. The body then takes all the excess it can't use and stores it as fat. So, on junk food and processed food, you not only become unhealthy because you gain weight, but on top of that, your body doesn't get all the vitamins, minerals, phytochemicals, and so on it needs to thrive. Add to that the possible disease causing chemicals that come in processed foods, and you can see how your body just can't win under these conditions.

It's not nearly as impossible to eat healthy as most people think. The more you eat of the right kinds of foods the more your taste buds start to wake up and enjoy them. You have to realize that processed food isn't real food and ditch it if you ever want to see any results that last. Forget about looking thin – get healthy first. Get rid of soft drinks, cookies, ice cream, candy bars, and anything with processed sugar. It's not the end of the world. People just don't know what they are missing in fruits and vegetables. There are so many great tasting, healthy, natural foods, like grapes, berries, apples, and yogurt, that can be eaten to replace a person's need for sweets. For protein, get chicken that doesn't have antibiotics that you cook yourself. You can add lemon juice and healthy spices for flavor, and you wind up eating tastier food than you ever thought possible while seeing physical results you couldn't imagine.

It is possible to go from flabby to fit and not have any superior genes or working out like they do on the reality TV shows. Most of our problem these days is what we eat and how much. Sure, you need to do more than sit all day, every day, but it doesn't take a supreme effort, like training for a Rocky movie, unless of course you aspire to look like a body builder. Then, yeah, you would need to hit the gym harder, but the average person would be amazed at how much their body would change by simply replacing processed foods that have all that excess sugar. It doesn't matter if you lift weights all the time for two hours a day, or just walk around the park every other day, you are going to see results and additional health benefits, if you don't take in processed sugary products.

There is no such thing as a magic diet that you do once that will give you a permanent perfect body. There's not even one you can do several times a year that has lasting effects. The only perfect diet is one that you follow on a daily and yearly basis for the rest of your life.

Diet plans are big business. There are tons of diet books and plans out there waiting to take your money. It cracks me up every time I see another magazine cover with claims of losing ten or twenty pounds in a month or week. First of all that's a pretty blanket statement that couldn't possibly cover everyone that reads the article. Everybody is different and everybody has a different body type and is at a different level of fitness or body fat ratio. If losing ten pounds is great for one person, it might mean becoming a stick figure for someone else. Diets should be about being healthy first and foremost. Believe me, all things being equal, the average person is going to see weight loss anyway once they get rid of junky garbage and sugar loaded processed foods. Don't spend any more money on special diets unless it's a diet that recommends healthy foods with lower sugar and fewer processed foods.

Then there's the person that starves for a while to lose weight. A low calorie starvation diet usually results in the dieter gaining more weight by the end of it because the dieter slows down his or her metabolism via the diet and then goes back to eating the same old fattening processed foods. A person will never succeed in losing weight and keep it off by going on a starvation diet. The key to weight loss is changing your lifestyle. It's about pursuing health for the long term. If you're not interested in having a healthy body, then you'll never have a trim, fit body either.

All those gimmicky infomercials showing the latest piece of exercise equipment are really annoying. Not because having exercise equipment is bad, because it's definitely not, but the commercials make it seem like all you have to do is a ten minute workout every day with their amazing new workout gadget and you'll look like a body builder in six weeks. They say nothing about diet other than maybe a footnote.

You have to have a little patience too. Losing weight the healthy way is often very gradual, but think of where you are now and where you can be in a year. Time goes by pretty fast, and in a year, a man or woman can see an amazing difference by cutting back on sugar and processed foods – and here's the important part – while adding healthy foods to take their place. Take in good carbs, like that which comes from fruit and vegetables, but get most of your carbs from green vegetables. Even too much fruit can be bad for your waist line, but, if it's a choice between apples and candy bars, go for the apples every time! And don't be afraid to eat beans a couple of times a week. Beans are a great source of fiber and nutrients and supply your carb needs. It's really hard to overeat fruits, vegetables and legumes thanks to the fiber that makes you feel full. It's God's way of keeping us from eating too much.

If this was just another diet plan, I'd call it the "Replacement Plan," but it's not just for a week or two, or even a month. It's the beginning of a lifestyle change.

The challenge is to find a healthier replacement for every food you buy. Here are some ideas:

Instead of potato chips, eat kale baked in the oven in coconut oil with a little added sea salt. It tastes great, and it's healthy.

Instead of soda, drink some tea. There are a lot of different flavors and varieties to choose from like herbal, white tea, or green tea. You can also squeeze some lemon or lime juice into your drink or add some stevia. Stevia is a much healthier choice than regular sugar or man-made sweeteners and it's very sweet to the taste. An important note though, people with ragweed allergies might also be allergic to stevia.

Instead of ice cream, try plain organic yogurt with added nuts, berries, unsweetened coconut flakes, and maybe a banana. Frozen mango tastes so good in yogurt you'll never need to eat ice cream again to satisfy your sweet tooth. There are a lot of different combinations you can go with here, but the end result should be tasty and filled with a lot of healthy nutrients. Plus the yogurt will help with digestion.

Instead of highly processed chicken nuggets, take some uncooked chicken tenders and add a little wheat germ, plus a few spices of your choice, and bake. It's a tasty treat with no harmful processed fat or sugar. Always avoid trans-fats that are found in some processed foods like the plague.

Instead of processed hamburger, cook some grass fed beef. It's got more vitamins and minerals than regular beef, and has more CLA which has been shown to trim a person's waist line over time.

Replace white bread with 100% whole wheat bread. I'm not big on eating too much of any bread, but whole wheat bread is a much better choice than white bread. It's best not to overdo wheat bread. I like to get most of my carbs from vegetables.

Use common sense when eating healthy fats, like avocados for example. They contain a lot of fat so I would recommend keeping it to one a day. There are limits to how much good fat a person can take in before gaining weight.

Organic popcorn is a great snack in place of regular popcorn. Pop it and add some light seasoning and skip the butter.

Do not buy junk food to take home with the idea that you'll just eat less. That never works. If you need to, let yourself have one bad food choice per shopping trip, but that's it. If you don't have it to eat at home, chances are you are not going to make a special trip to the grocery store to buy some junk food. If you do, that is a definite sign you are addicted to sugar and processed junk. The same principle works for cigarettes too, if you're a smoker. Don't buy it, and you can't smoke it. The hardest part of avoiding anything is that moment of temptation. If it's there with you all day or night then the temptation is there all day or night. If the temptation is only during a shopping trip, then you've got a much better chance of changing your life around for the better.

Surgery and Pills Verses Dietary Changes

Many people are opting for surgery these days to make the size of their stomachs smaller, after which they can only eat small portions at a time. This does help send signals to the brain that the stomach is full, but my concern is that if the person continues to eat the same types of foods, even in smaller amounts, they may eventually find themselves in as bad or worse shape physically than before. Sugar, even at small amounts, will just continue the cycle of insulin insensitivity. Thus, the person will start to gain weight again. Personally, while I do know a few people who have opted for surgery with success, I think it would be easier, and much healthier over the long haul, to first focus on creating new, healthy eating habits.

By surrounding yourself with only healthy food, eventually your system will correct itself, and you'll begin to enjoy those foods. Over time, as your body finally begins to gain all the nutrients it needs to sustain itself, you'll also feel more full and satisfied after a meal.

Our bodies need a certain amount of nutrients for energy; what they don't need is junk food and sugar. It's worthless to our bodies. Junk food goes to fat storage. Good food goes to energy and supplies the needs of all the activities that go on in our bodies from hair and skin maintenance to muscle growth and recovery.

When I was a teenager I lifted weights like I do now, but I couldn't understand why I never got as strong as I wanted to be. Now I know I could have been much stronger and so much further ahead, after years of working out, if I had just added a good diet to all that exercise I was doing.

People need to realize it isn't food in general that is the problem. It's sugar that causes a person to lose the ability to feel satisfied, which in turn makes them eat more and more. I was raised on sugary cokes and sweets, so if I can eat healthy anybody can. It's simply a matter of switching out processed junk food for healthy natural food.

Drinking fruit juice is not a good idea either, by the way. It has too much sugar, no fiber to fill you up, and, odds are, if it has been processed, it's had sugar added or other fake manmade sweeteners that have their own list of problems, weight gain being one of them.

Back to surgery, it's not really the easy option that people may believe. It comes with risks, is very painful, and the reason it works is that the person is forced to eat less because their stomach is smaller. Long term success isn't necessarily guaranteed, and there are some cases where the person made themselves sick by eating too much, despite the surgery. You can achieve the same goal of losing weight without all the pain by simply changing out junk food for good food. A person eating healthy food can still be thin and eat much larger portions than the tiny amounts allowed after surgery. Look at it this way, even after surgery you still need to eat healthy. Maybe even more so since you can only eat very small portions and your body still needs nutrients to function properly. Losing weight should be a result of being healthier not the result of starvation, and a body that doesn't get enough nutrients is starving.

I'm a firm believer that prevention is the safest way to go. Pills and surgeries should always be a last resort. These days doctors don't really take time to talk to their patients about living healthy. They are more likely to just hand their patient a prescription and show them the door. It seems that doctors are just less likely to preach healthy living and good prevention tips to their patients than in previous generations. Doctors are generally the focal point of pharmaceutical marketing campaigns. The pharmaceutical business is a business and its main concern is selling pills. Combine the sales tactics of drug companies with a society that wants a quick solution for every problem that doesn't require any discipline or extra work, and what you get is treatments that focus on symptoms rather than causes of illnesses.

Take those warnings seriously on the drug commercials. You know, the warnings that seem so outrageous that they are almost funny. It's not funny actually. The drug market doesn't want your doctor to prescribe you a diet of green vegetables to fix your ailments, not when they can sell you their handy dandy super treatment that only risks blindness, baldness, loss of limbs, and acute bleeding of the nose – oh, and sometimes death.

With all the problems associated with a poor diet, I wonder how many people realize it's likely that most of their health issues would go away if they would just change what they eat. The processed food we eat is not just junk, it's poison. But, how many doctors will take the time to tell their patients stop gorging on that poison and eat healthy?

I guess they don't have time to deal with unruly patients. It's just assumed no one has the willpower to make changes. So, even though, in most cases, dietary changes could not only save their patient a lifetime of prescription pills, not to mention the billions saved in the healthcare system overall nationwide, it's just too much trouble and aggravation for overworked doctors. Doctors today are increasingly overworked because of the number of patients created by our society's current lack of healthy lifestyle choices.

America was built on self-reliance, but right now she needs self-control more than anything. Too many people have equated not getting their way with suffering, and when it comes to food that could be extremely dangerous. Our grandfathers had to work hard for what they got. They knew the value of work and patience. They knew they couldn't always get what they wanted exactly when they wanted it. We need that kind of discipline today. Our "got to have it now" mentality hurts us financially and physically. The idea that there are no limits to our gratification has created a generation of obese children who suffer from diabetes, lack of mobility, not to mention the host of other issues down the road in life, and it's entirely our fault for not saying "no" occasionally.

Our kids think it's a sin, somehow, if we don't give them everything their heart desires when they want it. We need to teach them and ourselves to control what our heart desires, and not let our desires control us. I wonder how many families actually believe it's a sin almost not to pig out.

Portion Control

In the middle of the 2000's, Cornell researcher Brain Wasink performed an experiment called the "bottomless bowl of soup". He gave individuals self-filling bowls of tomato soup to see how they would naturally regulate how much they consumed. On average, they ate 73% more than control subjects with normal bowls. As this study shows, people have a tendency to keep eating as long as there is food in front of them. So, a good way to lose weight may sound overly simple, but just get smaller plates, bowls and cups, and don't order super-sized meals when you eat out. You can't necessarily rely on your appetite to tell you when to stop eating.

Some sources say that the average American is 26 pounds heavier than in the 1950s. The Centers for Disease Control and Prevention (CDC) says the average restaurant meal is now four times larger than it was in the 1950s.

One thing that has really changed since then, besides the lack of physical activity, is the portion sizes we eat. The size of a hamburger has tripled, a basket of fries more than doubled, and the average soda has grown from a modest 7 ounces to a jumbo 42 ounces. The very things that really add weight are the very items we eat more of than ever before, especially the fries and the soda.

Exercise

You might ask, "Why is exercise important?" Exercise reduces stress and cortisol release. Exercise increases muscle, improves cardiovascular functions, and improves endurance.

Get serious about your health. Start an exercise program to go with your new healthy diet. Exercise not only makes us healthier just by participating in it, it also helps us gauge our fitness level at the moment. If walking up the stairs leaves you winded, then you have a fair idea you are not as fit as you should be.

You can use your appearance as well as your physical abilities as a gauge as to where you are physically. Keep track of how much weight you can lift, how fast you can run or walk, how many repetitions of any particular exercise you can do and work on slowly improving in those areas. Weigh yourself daily to monitor any changes to your weight, and keep track of the size of your waistline.

It's not written in stone that as soon as you turn 40 all of your body parts are going to fall apart and you should look like you're one step away from the retirement home. Yes, we do get older, but it doesn't necessarily have to be nearly as fast as some people think. The problem is, people give up too easy. A man or woman that lives a healthy lifestyle should still be able to participate in his or her favorite sports, barring any serious injuries.

At 40, you might have to give up your dreams of ever playing in the NBA or the NFL, but the ability to run shouldn't be an impossible dream either; having said that, one does have to be careful to avoid injuries as we get older. An injury can hurt your ability to do basic exercises, but don't be afraid to move. Test yourself to see where you are physically.

A good way to burn fat and get your heart rate up is to lift weights, or do high intensity interval training (HIIT). You can do many variations of HIIT, but basically it involves moving as fast as you can for about 30 seconds, and then slowing down for a minute to a minute and a half. Repeat this cycle a total of six to ten times. You can use treadmills, indoor bikes, elliptical trainers, etc. for this type of program. You can even run/walk outside if you do not have access to any equipment. You'll just need a stopwatch. This type of workout is pretty intense, so you probably wouldn't want to do HIIT more than two to three times per week and make sure you warm up for about three to five minutes before you start.

Of course, if you haven't exercised in a long time, you should have a checkup with your doctor to make sure you are fit for exercise, but after that, start somewhere, even if it's just walking at the park or around your neighborhood. Walking is a great exercise for couples or for singles, but I find it particularly relaxing to walk and talk to my wife at the same time. In fact, I don't see how people sit still while talking. Walking helps me focus my thoughts.

With all the latest research pointing towards the fact that sitting for more than four hours a day, watching TV, playing games, or at the computer, can make a person twice as likely to have a cardiac event, I think we all should take up walking and talking in our leisure time. It's not going to blast away all of your fat in an hour, but it's natural. It's what God intended for us to do. He didn't intend for us to sit for hours every day the way we do in this modern day and time.

So play Frisbee. Get your family outside to play. There are a lot of relaxing ways to be active. Relaxing and moving do more than a couple of things for you at the same time. Stress is a killer deadlier than cigarettes. By moving, even if it's slowly, you burn more calories than sitting, and you keep blood flowing to all parts of your body.

Hard intense workouts make the muscles bigger, burn fat, and shape the body faster, but you can only do them so much during a week before you begin to overtrain. Overtraining is a condition where, instead of making your body healthier, you actually begin to lose strength and endurance. It's caused by working out harder and longer than your body can adapt to and recover from.

The best way to get in shape is by incrementally adding intensity or weight to your workouts every week. Beyond that, make exercise fun! The body and mind need to be constantly stimulated. Keep your body guessing as to what's coming up next. Change up the locations of your exercise. Take walks at different parks, or maybe go on a nature trail you've never been on before.

In terms of weightlifting, there are a thousand different workouts that build muscle. You can lift slowly to develop slow twitching muscle fibers, or go fast for fast twitching fibers. Do high numbers of repetitions with light weight, or go heavy with low reps for strength training. Don't get in a rut. The main thing is to always keep your workouts fun and interesting so that you can keep up your intensity level and motivation.

How to be Fat

Want to know how to be overweight and not even see it coming? Well, if you read this book, or anything else about diet and weight loss, you might not be surprised. But there are millions of people that are surprised that they've become fat over the years, eating what they considered to be average amounts of food.

People that work a lot and are always on the go tend to skip meals or replace them with chocolate bars, chips, crackers, and soft drinks until they can get home, but by that time they are starving and wind up eating a whole lot at once. This is a sure fire way to get huge and never see it coming.

Consuming sugar is the primary way to becoming overweight, even if it seems like you aren't eating that much. What you are eating goes straight to fat. The fact you haven't had a real meal all day makes it worse when you finally do eat. Your metabolism is slowed and your body stores everything it can for the next day. You basically train your body to hold onto everything. I have a friend that damaged his liver living off of sugar on the go. We see this happening more and more these days.

It may sound strange, but it's been proven that the more times you eat in a day the thinner you are likely to become, as long as you eat healthy foods. I bet you or somebody you know swears they eat hardly anything at all and yet they gain weight. This is because the few meals they do eat, they eat garbage, and the longer they wait between meals the slower their metabolism gets. It's a terrible cycle that makes people overweight, sometimes on very little food, and makes people think there is something wrong with them physically. There will be down the road, of course, if they don't correct their eating habits. Our bodies are trained by our lifestyles to either store food for long hauls, or burn it up for energy. Give your body good solid fuel on a regular basis and your body becomes an efficient fat burning machine with lots of extra energy and strength.

Make a Choice

Living healthy is all about making the right choices in life. Regardless of where you are physically you stand to gain from good healthy choices, whether it's eating right, being active, or quitting a bad habit, like smoking. I'm afraid a lot of people look at their weight and tell themselves they can't lose weight or become more physically fit.

There are some people that have real medical issues that will make it very difficult to lose weight. If you are truly overweight from years of eating junk food, then, logically, if you are now eating correctly and exercising at least 30 minutes to an hour a day, and still not losing weight, then you may need to see a doctor. It could be a sign something is wrong and that you need a doctor to examine you to find out what that might be. Weight issues could be a warning sign of something wrong physically, and not just an indication that the person is eating too much. It's always a good idea to pay attention to what is going on with our bodies.

People today, for the most part, are choosing to be overweight. Now, I'm sure somebody reading this is angry already. "What do you mean, I choose to be overweight? Of course I don't choose to be overweight, who would?" But what steps have you taken, I would ask that person. Have you started to write down everything you eat to hold yourself accountable? Have you started a workout plan for at least 30 minutes a day? You have to train yourself into good habits and then live that way to lose weight. As research has proven over and over again, simply going on a strict diet for a few weeks usually leads to more weight gained in the long run. It's how you live on a regular basis.

You have to permanently replace the bad foods with good foods you that can enjoy that don't leave you gaining weight every week or month. But listen, life is all about choices. As long as a person is aware of the health risks of being overweight, and as long as a person knows that basically they are choosing the joys of overindulging in ice cream, chips, and sodas over being fit and healthier, then that's fine. But I wonder if it registers with many Americans that the power to change is in their hands. It's not the government's choice to make you healthier. It's yours.

I hope I don't sound insensitive to folks that feel they can't help being overweight, but I know that if a person can get rid of junk food and stick to eating natural foods, like unprocessed meats, fruits, and vegetables, losing weight will happen, unless like I've said before you have a medical issue that you need to see a doctor about. It's not natural for people to have bellies that overlap their belts and hang toward the floor. A person has to admit that it's their choice to eat those cookies, and accept the consequences of their choice. We have power over what we eat or don't eat.

The victim mentality allows people to be overweight and not feel guilty. After all, if it's not your fault, then you and everybody else should just accept you at whatever lifestyle you choose to live, right? The problem is, no man or woman is an island, to coin a phrase. Our lives do affect others, especially our loved ones. People depend on us, and if our lives are cut short by bad choices, or we wind up in a hospital for things that could be avoided then we cause hurt, worries, and fears needlessly for those we love.

Trust me, I know life is hard, and it makes you want to do something, anything, to feel a little better. What could be so wrong about eating a bowl or two of ice cream for comfort after a rough day? Do you want the body of Stallone or the body of Wimpy the hamburger eater from the Popeye cartoons? Do you want to be healthy and have energy to do things now and further down the road? You have to judge your own actions as to how they are affecting your health. Nobody can do it for you. Being overweight isn't a sin, but gluttony is. Our bodies are basically organic machines, and they need maintenance and the right kind of fuel. Some people take better care of their cars than they do their own bodies. We owe it to God to be good stewards of everything He's given us, including our bodies.

We all have choices to make, and we all have our own roadblocks in the way of getting to our chosen goals. Life is like a rough boxing match sometimes. It will knock you on your butt and it will keep you there unless you get up and get up and get up again.

For the really motivated, if you can say to yourself I'd like to look like Stallone, the way he did in Rambo III, the movie he himself has said he was in the best shape of his life by the way, then all you got to do is ask question, "Do I choose to do that? Am I willing to pay the price?" Of course, the next thing you better ask is what is the price? Depending on what your goal is will determine the amount of exercise and the strictness of your diet. If all you want is to lose a few pounds and get relatively fit, then just start writing down all the food you eat in a week. Figure out how many calories and how much fat you took in, and then write down before you even go to the store what you need to buy to eat to replace those meals to get your calories down.

Look, if you decide for the first week not to worry about how much you eat, and just focus on what you eat, that's a huge step in the right direction. Just determine to replace each and every bad food choice you have. Ok, maybe you could let yourself have one thing per day, but only in moderation. That way you don't feel like you are suffering.

I tend to put my focus on eating healthy, period. I can tell if I eat too much from one day to the next without writing it down, but I've been at it for a while. It really helps to weigh yourself every day to get an idea of what foods cause you to gain or lose weight. If the average person eating 100 grams of sugar, or more, a day, probably more, would suddenly ditch the junk food in favor of real food, I could practically guarantee that the fat would come off and stay off as long as that person stays away from the junk food.

Doughnuts, cookies, ice cream, and cinnamon rolls have got to go. A box full of fried chicken isn't going to cut it either. Go green, eat kale and spinach, and even though I do recommend eating organic vegetables, if you are just starting out, just get whatever you can afford or get your hands on that's a fruit or vegetable. It's better to buy conventional produce than to buy processed junk foods. It might have pesticides, but then processed foods are made of foods that contain pesticides too, before all the other garbage is added

Eating foods like spinach, mushrooms, lentils, beans, asparagus, broccoli, and kale is a sure fire way to lose weight. The fiber is going to fill you up. Your stomach is going to feel like it's pumped full of air, but that's good. A belly filled with fiber is less likely to grow more fat attached to it.

For snacks, you dine on apples, nuts, berries, bananas, carrots, avocados. You want to keep these otherwise healthy foods down to one a day. The sugar in fruits has to be kept to a minimum, and the fat in one avocado is a lot, even though it's the healthy kind of fat, your body can process more easily. More than one a day is going to push you over the limit.

Get some white meat chicken breasts, and a little bit of hamburger, grass fed if you can afford it. Eggs are great too. You need plenty of protein especially if you are working out like you should be.

Just sit down and brainstorm all the healthy foods a person can buy, write it down, and then stock your fridge and cabinets full. If you still have to overeat, let it be healthy food at least. You'll eventually start to lose weight once your body starts to regulate your appetite to where it should be.

Here's another thing to remember, healthy food is tasty, and if you take the time to cook it yourself and prepare your meals ahead of time for work, you will ultimately enjoy your meals more in the long run. Junk food has a tendency to ruin our taste buds to real food. Remember rat poison tastes good to rats. So just because you believe junk food is great tasting, that doesn't mean you should eat it.

I love chicken breast with some freshly squeezed lemon juice poured on top as it cooks. Of course, some herbs and spices go a long way to making food taste good and even add more health benefits.

Getting into shape can be fun if you choose it to be. If you choose to only enjoy garbage food, then that's all you will ever enjoy. If you choose to love wholesome good food then you will.

Here's something to think about, the Bible teaches that love is a choice. We are commanded to love God with all our hearts. We can choose to love or hate the right kinds of foods. We are what we choose to be and what we choose to love. Growing up, I literally chose to hate healthy food. I thought of salads as being the same as eating grass, so I can relate to people who have a hard time changing from junk food to real food.

There are a lot of Americans out there today that are choosing to believe that processed foods are somehow better than real food, when processed foods start out as real food before chemicals and preservatives are added and before the mixing and mashing together is done. Hot dogs start from real meat, but who knows what it is by the time they get done with it. Have you ever read the ingredients to potted meat? They actually put mashed animal tongues in potted meat. Who knows, that might be a delicacy in some places, but for some reason it's not something I care for.

Sometimes we gravitate towards certain foods and activities because of experiences we've had growing up, but you can grow up in a family that eats perfectly every day of the week and still decide that's not for you.

I hope in some small way this book can convince those on the fence to choose healthy foods. There are so many new people every day who are wind up sick and in the hospital. Wouldn't it be nice if even a small percentage of cancers, heart problems, and general illnesses could be stopped in their tracks, or at the very least put off until later in life, by simple healthy lifestyle changes? There really is a lot more at stake than just losing a few pounds, as important as that is.

But, again, do research and look on the internet for healthy foods, and write down the foods in this book that are healthy that you might like before you even go into a store. Sometimes you can't find everything you want, so you need some backup choices just in case.

But do not buy fruit juice thinking it's healthy. The vitamins might make it healthier than cokes, but the sheer volume of sugar in a fruit juice drink is not worth it. The biggest weapon you have in your arsenal of weight loss is avoiding sugary drinks and replacing them with water or tea. You do not want to drink cokes or sugary drinks if you are choosing to lose weight and be healthy. It will not work. Soft drinks have got to go first if a person is serious about losing fat, and keeping it off.

6 MAKING THE RIGHT HABITS

Being fit and healthy in the long run and reaching your full potential in the gym, and in your physique, is going to depend on making good habits in life. It doesn't matter if you are way overweight, really thin, or have been religiously working out for your entire life, making new or additional good habits, and breaking old bad habits, are key to reaching your health goals. If you don't have any goals, then making goals should be the first step. A person without goals is just shooting in the dark hoping to hit something, but they're not sure what.

Make short-term and long-term goals. The short-term, easier goals are to help keep you motivated and encouraged as you go along toward your ultimate fitness goals. Now that you have set your goals ask yourself, "What is keeping me from reaching my first short term goal?" It might be something major like smoking, or it might be something smaller like just a little bit too much sugar or carbs in your diet. Whatever it is, pinpoint it, and eliminate it.

It may be that you need more activity. Sometimes your normal workout isn't enough to reach your weight loss goals, and yet you might feel that you couldn't work out any harder without risk of overtraining. Our bodies are not made to sit, so you might consider making a habit of going for a walk around your neighborhood or at the park on the weekends or in the evenings with your spouse. Walking is therapeutic. It keeps the blood flowing in your body, and it helps the body heal faster from a hard workout.

If you don't work out at all, then it's a no-brainer – you need to get into the habit right now. You know your schedule, work it in somewhere and do it the same time every day. Even if you only have ten minutes, you can work miracles in ten minutes a day if you slowly increase the intensity of the workout over time. Sure, I highly recommend a little longer than that, but if a person can just spare twenty minutes a day, they should be able to get enough exercise to build muscle and lose weight. Keep in mind, though, the battle for your physique is won with your diet. It only takes a few minutes of exercise a day to make a difference, but eating comes up all day long.

The next habit is planning out your meals for the next day. Think about what you are going to eat ahead of time. A body builder might want to map meals out for a whole week so they can have a high-carb day, and a low-carb day, and relate all of it to their workout schedule.

Get in the habit of preparing your food for the next day and taking it to work with you. If you don't have food with you, you will most likely end up eating processed junk from some restaurant on your lunch break, or worse, hitting the vending machines for sugary snacks. Don't let yourself get hungry. That leads to temptation. Have healthy snacks ready to go to eat right before you start to get hungry. Nip your bad cravings in the bud with some nuts, maybe some tuna, an apple, etc. You get the point. A person who isn't prepared will fall victim to whatever junk food or processed garbage they can get their hands on at the time.

If you sit at desk job all day, get into a habit of standing up as often as possible. I don't care if you lift weights like Arnold and Sly after work; it's not healthy to sit still in one place for 8-10 hours a day. More and more research shows that no matter how much a person exercises, long stretches of continuous sitting makes them more prone to a cardiac event.

Make a habit of tracking your food over the course of a day. Lots of websites offer their members the ability to track the food they eat, and get nutritional information about the foods in their diet.

Don't forget to make good spiritual habits as well, like reading your Bible and praying every day. You can starve to death spiritually if you don't read enough of God's Word. As Christians, we all know that our spiritual attitudes can change very easily for the worse when we forget to read the Bible on a daily basis. Think about how irritable and weak you get when you skip a meal, and then consider the spiritual consequences to our hearts and Christian walk with God when we skip our spiritual food.

Keep up with health news at sites like our hip2bfit.com. It always pays to know what's going on in the latest health studies.

Avoiding Bad Habits

Smoking

Obviously, one of the worst habits to be in is a cigarette habit. It's a dangerous game people play hoping or just choosing to believe it's the other guy that will get cancer or heart disease, but not me. I actually used to smoke, so I know how addictive nicotine is. I was probably a bigger idiot about smoking than most people. Back in my twenties, I would actually be in the middle of workout in the gym, and then go outside to puff a cigarette. Oh, and then I wondered why I felt dizzy. It's not one of my prouder moments in logical thinking, but is there ever really a time when smoking a cigarette is smart? It also illustrates how folks that smoke tend to look at smoking as something akin to drinking water as if it were a necessity to life instead of a hindrance.

What infuriates me is the notion that cigarette companies have actually gone out of their way to make cigarettes more addictive over the years. They definitely have not been working to make cigarettes healthier. No, their goal has been to manufacture, basically, the perfect people trap. They get their customers addicted and hope they beat the odds long enough to keep them buying their product. It should make smokers angry that they are being taken advantage of this way.

Do you know that rat poison is one of the ingredients in cigarettes? How is it sane to sell rat poison for people to inhale?

Facts about Smoking

Statistics indicate that adult smokers can expect to take a minimum of 14 years off their lives.

Cigarettes are so addictive that up to 70 percent of smokers would like to quit, but have been unsuccessful.

A Massachusetts law forcing tobacco companies to report test results has shown that the tobacco industry has been making cigarettes more addictive.

Between 1998 and 2004, manufacturers increased the amount of addictive nicotine by 10 percent.

Smoking, or exposure to cigarette smoke, can be linked to an increased risk of hearing loss according to one study.

A Canadian study has suggested that it may take only one cigarette for some people to become addicted to nicotine.

Cigarettes contain over 4,000 different chemicals, all with varying degrees of toxicity.

The American Cancer Society reported that smoking cigarettes kills more Americans than alcohol, car accidents, suicide, AIDS, homicide, and illegal drugs combined.

There are so many toxic chemicals in cigarettes that some are using the term third hand smoking to describe the issues surrounding children coming into contact with chemical mess that stays around a smoker's hair, clothes, furniture, etc.

Tobacco is the sixth highest out of all agricultural crops in terms of the amount of pesticides applied per acre, the General Accounting Office and CBS News reported.

The pesticides used in tobacco production have been linked to cancer, nervous system damage and birth defects.

Some of the chemicals found in tobacco smoke might shock you – like acetone, also used in nail polish remover, acetic acid, also found in hair dye, ammonia, arsenic used in rat poison, benzene used in rubber cement, cadmium found in battery acid. I mean, come on, rat poison and battery acid, if that's not enough to make you want to quit, then you know cigarettes have gotten a terrible hold on you. If that's not enough, there are also chemicals found in rocket fuel, lighter fluid, embalming fluid, material used to pave roads, and one used to make paint.

Smoking may diminish the speed and accuracy of your thinking and reduce your IQ.

An estimated 50,000 Americans lose their lives to secondhand smoke annually.

A history of smoking on a daily basis is a risk factor for development of major depression.

Research has shown that cigarettes are contaminated with bacteria. This may explain why smokers' respiratory tracts tend to contain higher levels of disease-causing bacteria. Of course, this may also be a symptom caused by weakened immunity, which is also common in smokers.

Smoking causes wrinkles by upsetting the body's mechanism for renewing skin. Smoking disrupts the body's natural process of breaking down old skin and renewing it. It's bad enough to die early, but the fact is, cigarettes make us appear much older than we are.

The University Of Minnesota Division Of Periodontology reports that smoking is as addictive as heroin. Seriously, can a person justify a habit that has anything in common with heroin?

Children who grow up with smokers in their homes are three times more likely to develop lung cancer in their later years than those children who come from non-smoking homes. This one really gets me because it shows just how addictive cigarettes are. When I was a smoker I ignored second hand smoke warnings thinking they were just politically correct garbage. I didn't realize, until after I had done tons of research, just how dangerous chemicals in common every day household items in general can be, much less those that are found in second hand smoke. It's so much easier to dismiss these warnings than to have to face what a person's smoking might be doing to their kids and those around them. I wish somebody would have hit me over the head with the facts a long time before I actually quit. If you smoke, please don't ignore the warnings. It's one thing to smoke if you believe it just hurts you, but it really does hurt the health of your family as well. Besides, even if second hand or even third hand smoke wasn't a reality, do you have the right to deprive your loved ones of your presence before your time has come? What about the medical bills?

How I Quit

Like I've mentioned, I know how hard it is to quit smoking. It's not easy at all. Personally, I credit my quitting to answered prayer, but before a person quits they have to fully understand the consequences of smoking. They have to come to themselves and let it fully sink in. You have to truly want to quit before you can even say a prayer to quit, and most smokers do not really want to quit until they face the full consequences of smoking.

Fortunately, for me my long term goals have always been centered around being in shape. I've worked out in a gym since I first got a driver's license back in my teens. I never really quite understood in my younger years though, how living a healthy lifestyle was essential to getting stronger or looking fit. I was stuck on the idea that I could overcome any health obstacle by simply working out harder. Of course, nothing could be further from the truth. You don't put garbage into your car's gas tank and expect to get much out of it.

As I got older, I started to have a few issues on top of never making much progress in the gym. This eventually led to eating healthier and spending hours upon hours researching what is healthy and what is not, but the first thing to be tackled in my life was cigarettes. I prayed about quitting for years, but never could beat it. I began to become more desperate to quit and so I spent hours researching what cigarettes actually do to the body. The more you know about the harmful effects of smoking, the more you can build up the desire necessary to quit. I must have quit and started back dozens of times, but slowly and surely the thought started to enter my mind, "Keep smoking and you are going to die". It wasn't simply paranoia. I'd seen how close to dying members in my family had gotten, not to mention the ones that had died already from smoking.

Smoking wasn't worth it; I knew that, but why couldn't I quit? Finally, I did quit for the very last time. I knew cutting back wasn't going to work. It had to be completely gone out of my life. Before, I would keep a pack lying around for emergencies, even though as a Christian I should have been relying on Jesus for whatever might come into my life, not lifeless smoke from a cigarette to get through problems.

I hate to say it, but I almost cried the day I quit, as if I'd lost a friend. Yes, cigarettes are insanely addictive. That fact alone should make a smoker mad enough to fight it with everything they have. No addictive substance has ever been good for anything.

After that final day I never lit another cigarette, after so many failed attempts at cutting back, and quitting, and starting again. This time it was if God flipped a light switch in my brain, and I knew my days of smoking were over.

So, if you smoke and you really want to quit, prayer is very effective, but God doesn't make anybody do anything they don't really want to do. So face the consequences of smoking. Make health goals and keep at it, realizing it has to stop. You cannot be right in your mind and put your life and the lives of those around you at risk, for what, a puff of smoke that you can never get your hands around. Smoking never satisfies. The more you smoke the more you want to smoke.

Also, to help you quit, reward yourself with fun activities – as long as it's not junk food. Go walking, play sports, go to the gym, keep busy while you are going through withdrawals. If possible, take a vacation during the first week you quit. Avoid stress if at all possible.

What Happens After Quitting

It's amazing what happens after you quit smoking. I even dreamed about cigarettes at first. But after a month or two I didn't think about it anymore, during the day at least. Occasionally, I still do dream about smoking, but just as a nightmare. These days, the nightmare goes that I've started again after all this time. You see, I know that if I were to have that one cigarette I could potentially start the addiction process all over again. So, it goes without saying that as a cigarette addict, I know I can't be hanging around people that smoke. This is why cutting back may be an ok way to start the process of quitting, but eventually you have to go to a no tolerance policy for cigarettes. You can't have them around you. This is one reason why I imagine it's nearly impossible for people to quit in homes that have more than one smoker. Timing the quitting process simultaneously must be extremely difficult, especially given the anger and stress that comes with quitting during the first few weeks.

Eventually, except for the occasional bad dream, it becomes like you never smoked at all. Funny thing, I know a person's ability to smell increases because I can smell a smoker a mile away now. I can walk outside and know if a smoker has been by that vicinity recently.

Physically, your body starts to heal itself even after only one day has passed from the day you quit smoking. The chances of having a heart attack actually decrease in 24 hours. Withdrawal symptoms reach their peak within 48 to 72 hours. Within three months, your circulation will improve and your lung function will increase by as much as 30%.

The best thing about completely getting rid of smoking from your life is that you actually feel less stressed. The biggest excuse I had to keep smoking was that my nerves were bad and somehow the cigarettes were these magical wonder sticks that made me feel all better. The problem with that thinking was the cravings for the cigarettes every two hours were what was causing me to be nervous in the first place. I'm not the calmest person in the world, even today, but not having intense cravings for nicotine makes me a much more stable, happy person. If you smoke now, know that it will make you a more relaxed and happier person when you quit smoking too, once you get over the cravings.

For Christians, quitting smoking really is a no brainer. The Bible says, "Thou shalt have no other gods before me". Smoking's incredible addictive nature is so powerful it can't be considered anything else but a god in our lives. Think about it, anything that a person would trade for their very health and the health of their families has become more important to that person than God in their lives. The same can be said of junk food when it starts to rob a person of their health. I personally believe sugar can also be an idol in a Christian's life. Read more about sugar and it's addictive nature in Chapter 4.

How to Beat a Soft Drink Addiction

Want to lose weight and keep it off? Then the very first step you need to take is to stop drinking soft drinks and even what some might consider healthy, fruit juice drinks that have just about as much or more sugar than soft drinks. Getting rid of soft drinks also rids you of a major source of fat producing sugar and calories. Everyone can benefit from replacing soft drinks in their daily lives, whether you are fighting obesity, are just a little overweight, or trying to get that ripped look. Even avid weight lifters and runners should avoid sodas for better performance in their workouts. Not only can getting rid of sugary drinks help you athletically, it can also help get you ripped for those that just need to cut out a few more pounds.

Over time, the pounds you can lose from ditching sugar filled drinks can really add up. You'll see a huge difference. Plus the inflammation soft drinks create isn't good for anyone's health long term. As we get older we start to feel the aches and pains of life, and the last thing anyone needs is body inflaming sugar. Getting rid of sugar could drastically improve a person's ability to exercise, and to get around in general, by decreasing inflammation, and, therefore, pain as well. It would probably be shocking to find out how many people suffer from chronic back pain and other ailments because of the sugar they get every day just in their drinks alone.

I need to point out that soft drinks and processed sugary drinks and food are addictive. It's not the kind of addiction that society or the church looks down on, like cigarette smoking or alcoholism, but the sad thing people don't realize is that sugar addiction is just as dangerous as those other addictions, and, for some people, can be even worse.

The biggest source of sugar for the average person these days is soft drinks, and they can be difficult to give up, but not impossible. I used to drink several cokes a day myself, back before I woke up to the fact that weight lifting and cardio alone wasn't all I needed to be healthy. I was practically raised on soft drinks. I guess my parents didn't see the harm in it, and when you are younger, you can get away with it, or so it seems, if you are very active, the way kids used to be, at least. Of course, sugar causes internal health issues not necessarily seen on the outside right away. But these days, with the lack of activity accompanied by an increased sugar intake, we see the effects more readily on kids and adults.

Even if you are very active you can reap great benefits by ditching the soft drink habit. Sugar causes inflammation, which is the enemy of health and can really hold you back in the gym. To put it into perspective, one canned soft drink exceeds the amount of sugar you should typically consume in one entire day and then some. Just one soda a day will make you continuously gain weight over the course of a year.

Once I quit drinking soft drinks, I lost weight gradually and have kept it off without much extra effort. Sugar sabotages a person's efforts to lose weight. I think a lot of the fat we attribute to being older has more to do with soft drinks and other sources of processed sugar. Assuming you agree and really want to make that change in your life for a healthier thinner you, here are some tips for ditching the soft drink habit. One more thing though - diet drinks are no better. Studies show those drinking diet drinks gradually gain even more weight than those drinking the real thing. Basically remember, if it's not natural, its suspect.

My Tips for Replacing Soft Drinks

When you are ditching some bad habit in your life, it makes it much easier if you can replace it with something good.

Teas

Tea is my favorite drink these days. Growing up I couldn't stand the stuff, but I never knew there were so many different flavors to choose from.

Brew your own. Do not buy the processed kind with sugar already added. Tea not only can be a tasty replacement for soft drinks, but it's good for you. It's filled with antioxidant properties and phytochemicals that may help prevent cancer depending on the type of tea you drink. To get the most health benefits, the caffeinated varieties, like green teas have the most bang for your buck. In general, tea contains catechins, a type of antioxidant. Catechins are highest in concentration in white and green teas.

1. To make tea fun to drink, try the all the various flavors, like green tea with pomegranate, or other various berry flavors. There are also lots of non-caffeinated herbal teas in a variety of flavors to try like blueberry, cherry, raspberry, wild berry, and on and on and on.

2. Now, if you need some added flavor, try squeezing the juice from a lemon or lime, in which the sugar and fructose content is very low, into your glass.

3. Still need more sweetness? Try stevia; it's completely natural and doesn't have all the bad effects of the fructose or all the chemicals found in soft drinks.

There are many teas to try, so don't assume that, because you do not like straight up green tea, you won't like all the rest.

Lemon and/or Lime Water
1. Just as you can add a little lemon or lime, or both, to your tea, you can also add it to just plain water for a great, fun, healthy drink.

2. Again, if you really need a sweet drink, add some stevia, but personally I don't like to overdo it. I try to keep it to one or two packs of stevia a day. Sometimes I use two to four packs for an entire jug of tea, for instance. Be aware though, if you add stevia, there are some people that have allergies to stevia.

Water

There is nothing better for you in the world than just plain water. I recommend getting a filter and making tap water high on your list. Eventually, you'll lose the taste for soft drinks, and seriously you figure out that life does not revolve around sugary drinks, especially once you figure out the high cost of soft drinks to your body and your bank account.

Don't Bring it Home

Here's what I did when I was quitting cokes. I told myself I could have a coke whenever I wanted one, just not at home. Now, I work from home so it's a little different for me. If you drink soft drinks all day at work, this isn't going to help you, but the basic idea is to not bring soft drinks home, even if you have to spend more for those smaller containers. It's about making that Coke or Pepsi a special event like for a Christmas party or a trip to town on the weekend. It's good to remember that soft drinks will still be there; you don't have to panic. After a while you will lose your taste for soft drinks and you'll never miss them. Heaven forbid, you might actually prefer the taste of water, in time, to that chemical soup mix of sugar and syrup we call soft drinks.

Bottom Line

Cutting out soft drinks is likely, for most Americans, the biggest and fastest change that can be made to improve their overall health in a short time, assuming that smoking isn't a problem in that person's life. There really isn't any excuse not to quit when there are so many tasty varieties of tea on the market. It's all a matter of taking the time to find the flavors that you like. So, it might take a little effort to brew verses an already made coke. A little effort goes a long ways toward saving your life. I mean, would you drink rat poison if someone added enough sugar? I've heard that arsenic actually tastes sweet, so remember taste can be deceiving.

7 SUPER FOODS

In this section we will look at what I like to think of as super foods. These are foods that taste great and have great nutritional value. They are foods that won't add to your waist line. It is very important for your fitness goals to replace bad food with good, whether you've been working out for years, or have just gotten serious about diet and exercising. As important as exercise is, you can't beat poor nutrition with exercise alone. Processed food and sugar are anchors holding you down and keeping you from moving forward toward your fitness goals.

One thing to remember about food verses supplements is that foods have various phytochemicals that are thought to lower the risk of cancer, among other health benefits, that just aren't available in vitamin supplements.

Apples

Apples are at the top of the list for healthy foods, if you eat the organic variety. This is one healthy food that you want to stay clear of in the conventional produce section. Unfortunately, it's one fruit that is always listed as having more pesticides than most other fruits.

Medium sized apples have about 4 grams of fiber and only about 95 calories. Apples are also a great source of vitamin C. Many studies indicate that apples may help prevent cancer, control sugar problems, help prevent heart disease, lower cholesterol, provide anti-inflammatory protection, and help promote weight loss. Apples contain phytonutrients, like quercetin.

Don't forget an apple a day keeps the doctor a way. Just make it an organic apple.

Asparagus

Asparagus is high in folic acid and a good source of potassium, fiber, thiamin, and vitamins A, B6, E, K, and C. It also contains iron, phosphorus, potassium, copper, manganese, chromium, and selenium. It can be cooked or eaten raw. Don't be alarmed if your urine has an unusual odor after eating asparagus. This is temporary and perfectly natural and has even sparked various studies.

Avocado

Avocados are one of my favorites. The fruit has a lot of healthy, monounsaturated fat that is easily burned for energy, but it is still fat so I recommend having no more than one serving per day. It's very low in fructose, which is the bad part of sugar and what you want to avoid as much as possible. Avocados are high in fiber, have more potassium than a banana, and they promote heart health. They are also rich in B vitamins, as well as vitamin E and vitamin K. Their thick skin protects the fruit from pesticides, making them a good option for those who want to avoid cancer causing chemicals without having pay extra for organic.

The best thing about avocados is that they taste great. I love to add some tuna, a few crackers, and maybe a hardboiled egg for a super snack. I wouldn't recommend eating avocado before or directly after a workout, however. The high fat content makes it hard to process during a high activity period. Make sure you have plenty of time to digest before a workout and also be aware some people do have allergies to avocados.

Do not eat avocados at night because you will gain weight and you might wind up with a little heartburn overnight. I've found for me, the best time to eat avocados is somewhere between 12 and 4.

Bananas

Bananas are an excellent source of vitamin B6, manganese, and potassium. I usually only eat one banana a day, in my daily yogurt snack, so I can keep my sugar intake as low as possible; however, a banana is a good choice for a healthy balanced diet. One large banana can pack a little over 600 mg of potassium, two grams of protein and four grams of fiber, and only carry 140 calories. A banana also has vitamin A and a full range of B vitamins including thiamine, riboflavin, niacin, vitamin B6, and folic acid. Bananas also contain vitamin C with minerals calcium and magnesium, and trace amounts of iron and zinc.

Beans

Beans are a healthy source of protein, B vitamins, iron, magnesium, potassium, copper, and zinc. They have loads of antioxidants and are an excellent source of fiber. Eating beans regularly may decrease the risk of diabetes, heart disease, colorectal cancer, and help with weight management. The dried beans you have to cook yourself pack the most antioxidants and nutrients compared with the canned varieties. Canned beans also have a lot of sodium and other potentially harmful chemicals or additives.

There are several varieties of red beans including small red beans, red kidney beans and adzuki beans. Red beans come out on top of lists for the most antioxidants alongside wild blueberries. Small red beans and kidney beans can have over 13,000 antioxidants per serving. Red beans are low on the glycemic index, which makes them good for stabilizing blood sugar levels. According to the Mayo Clinic, consuming red kidney beans may help prevent the occurrence of chronic diseases such as heart disease and cancer.

Beef

Grass fed beef is a much healthier choice than the conventional grain fed beef. It is, unfortunately, at this time, more expensive than the conventional beef. Grass fed beef is lower in saturated fats, slightly higher in omega 3 fatty acids, and higher in CLA which studies have shown can help a person obtain a smaller waist line. Grass fed beef is also higher in vitamins A and E.

Berries

Blueberries

Blueberries contain vitamins A and C, zinc, potassium, iron, calcium and magnesium, are high in fiber and low in calories, and are packed with phytochemicals.

Research has shown that blueberries contain pterostilbene, anthocyanins, proanthocyanidins, resveratrol, flavonols, and tannins, which inhibit cancer cell development and inflammation in the body.

USDA Human Nutrition Center (HNRCA) has ranked blueberries number one in antioxidant activity.

Blueberries are thought to help many health issues including possibly alleviating the cognitive decline occurring in Alzheimer's, help with urinary tract infections, and help with memory. One study using rats showed the rats fed blueberry extract were smarter than rats on a standard diet.

One nice attribute found was that blueberries may help you lose the belly fat and help with diabetes. In a study using rats, after 90 days, rats that received a blueberry-enriched diet had less abdominal fat, lower triglycerides, lower cholesterol, and improved fasting glucose and insulin sensitivity. I love to have blueberries almost every day with my nightly yogurt snack.

The one downside to blueberries is that you **do** want to buy organic, as conventional blueberries have a lot of pesticides used in farming.

Cranberries

Cranberries are best known for as a treatment for urinary tract infections. Cranberries are rich in polyphenols, which are potent antioxidants. Research indicates that cranberries may lower cholesterol and help fight against cancer. You'll notice a lot of what you read about fruits and vegetables is that they help fight cancer while on the other hand junk food more likely is thought to cause cancer, heart disease, and other diseases.

Raspberries

Raspberries are rich in anthocyanins and cancer-fighting phytochemicals such as ellagic, coumaric and ferulic acid. They also contain calcium, vitamins, such as A, C, and E, fiber, and folic acid. Raspberries also help lower cholesterol. They have also been shown to protect against certain kinds of cancer.

Strawberries

Strawberries rank right under blueberries for their amount of antioxidant punch. They contain fiber and manganese, and contain more vitamin C than any other berry. Their antioxidants are anthocynanins and ellagic acid, a phytochemical that has been shown to fight carcinogens. It's a good idea to buy organic strawberries to avoid pesticides.

Broccoli

Broccoli is loaded with vitamins. It's high in vitamin C and contains fiber for digestion. It also has the highest levels of carotenoids in the brassica family. It is particularly rich in lutein and also provides beta-carotene. Broccoli also contains vitamin E, K, calcium, iron, magnesium, phosphorus, potassium, zinc, and B vitamins.

The 3,3'-Diindolylmethane found in broccoli is a potent modulator of the innate immune response system with anti-viral, anti-bacterial and anti-cancer activity.

Broccoli can be boiled, steamed, or eaten raw. Boiling reduces the levels of suspected anti-cancer compounds in broccoli, with losses of 20 – 30% after five minutes, 40 – 50% after ten minutes, and 77% after thirty minutes. Steaming broccoli for 3–4 minutes is recommended to maximize potential anti-cancer compounds, such as sulforaphane.

Broccoli also has indole-3-carbinol, a chemical which boosts DNA repair in cells and appears to block the growth of cancer cells. Broccoli is said to decrease the risk of prostate cancer and heart disease.

Celery

A one cup serving of celery provides 37 percent daily value of vitamin K, 9.1 percent DV both of folate and vitamin A, 5.2 percent DV of vitamin C, 3.7 percent DV vitamin B6, 3.4 percent DV vitamin B2, and small amounts of a variety of other vitamins. Celery's mineral list from a one cup serving includes 7.5 percent potassium, 5.2 percent manganese, and 4 percent calcium.

Celery has flavonoids, which may lower the risk of cancer, inflammatory and cardiovascular diseases. Phthalides found in celery are thought to lower stress by regulating stress hormones and may improve blood flow.

Celery makes a great snack, as a cup of celery contains only 16 calories and only .2 gram of fat. Celery contains about 1.6 grams of sugar, which isn't bad at all for a snack. Try a few stalks with a tablespoon of nut butter or hummus.

Chicken Breast

Chicken breast is the favorite food for body builders as it is a great source of lean protein. It contains niacin, vitamin B-6, and selenium. Selenium is a trace mineral that supports immunity, promotes healthy thyroid function and may offer protection against cancer and heart disease.

If you can afford it, I highly recommend starting with fresh or frozen raw organic chicken breasts if you want to avoid all the additives and the antibiotics that conventional chicken contains. Sometimes you can find it at about the same price as the conventional chicken.

There are a couple of things I like to do with chicken. First, you can squeeze fresh lemon juice onto it as soon as you start cooking it to let it absorb into the meat. I like to use coconut oil for cooking.

Another great choice to cook your chicken in is organic steak sauce. I actually like to mix the two, but try it both ways to see what you prefer. There shouldn't be more than a couple of grams of sugar per serving in the steak sauce.

If you really want to go for a super lightweight meal for weight loss, for a side choose something like broccoli, cauliflower, carrots, or mushrooms. Of course there are many spices to choose from to add flavor. Cook it slow and put some time into it, and you'll never miss processed chicken again. It is a good idea to cook a little extra for later on. It saves time, and it's great to take to work the next day.

Dark Chocolate

Dark chocolate can be a great healthy treat and might help keep your cravings for sweets under control. It is a potent antioxidant, but you should limit yourself to one small piece per day. Eat more than that and the health consequences can quickly start to outweigh the benefits, thanks to the sugar and inevitable weight gain overeating dark chocolate can cause.

One thing to keep in mind is that milk may interfere with the absorption of antioxidants from chocolate which would negate the health benefits of eating dark chocolate. So milk chocolate, or washing dark chocolate down with a glass of milk, is not the healthiest option.

Dark Chocolate may even have a healthy effect on your teeth. Here's the thing though, if you don't think you can keep it to just one very small piece a day, then, for the sake of your waistline, this is one super food you might want to pass on.

Eggs

Eggs are a great health food for the average family. They are easy to fix, and cheap, which makes them great for the family on a budget. I do encourage you to spend just a little more for the cage free variety, at least, and for the best nutrient capacity get the organic cage free eggs. Chickens that are put into small cages are not nearly as healthy and they of course produce eggs that aren't as healthy for humans to eat. It's really common sense when you think about it. How healthy do you think you'd be in a small cage all your life? The free range chickens have better diets and this also gives hens the ability to lay healthier eggs for human consumption.

For a while we were told not to eat eggs because the cholesterol would cause us to have heart attacks, but that conventional wisdom has changed. It's again healthy to eat eggs. No, the egg didn't change, but doctors and scientists are now finding out that dietary cholesterol doesn't cause high blood cholesterol, as was previously believed.

Here are some the things you'll find in an egg including several vitamins and minerals like vitamin A, vitamin B2, vitamin B9, vitamin B6, vitamin B12, choline, iron, calcium, phosphorus and potassium. They are also a great source of protein.

All of the egg's vitamins A, D, and E are in the egg yolk. The egg is one of the few foods that naturally contains vitamin D. The egg yolk was supposed to be the bad part that we weren't supposed to eat, but by throwing it away, we lost out on all those vitamins.

A large yolk contains more than two-thirds of the recommended daily intake of 300 mg of cholesterol. One study, however, has indicated the human body may not absorb much cholesterol from eggs anyway, but this is something to keep in mind if you are on a low cholesterol diet.

Egg yolk also contains choline, which is an important nutrient for development of the brain, and is said to be important for pregnant and nursing women to ensure healthy fetal brain development. Choline is the precursor molecule for the neurotransmitter acetylcholine, which is involved in many functions including memory and muscle control. Choline is essential for the body to remain healthy. It is found in other healthy foods as well, like almonds, spinach, quinoa, peanuts, chicken, milk, and kidney beans.

More and more studies emerge that support the egg's importance in a good, balanced diet. In fact, I read about one recent study said that those that ate eggs for breakfast stayed satisfied longer, which adds up to eating less in the long run. Food that takes care of your nutritional needs satisfies the body in general. Junk food only makes you hungrier because the body doesn't get what it needs.

Eggplant

One cup of diced eggplant contains approximately two percent of the recommended dietary allowance of vitamin C and one percent of vitamin A, calcium and iron. Eggplant also contains four percent of the RDA for vitamin K, the vitamin that helps with blood clotting. It also provides six percent of the RDA for manganese, which acts as an antioxidant to help with wound healing and bone health. Eggplant contains the antioxidant nasunin which may be good for preventing cellular damage in the brain. Eggplants are also high in a chlorogenic acid, a powerful antimicrobial and antiviral antioxidant that has the ability to help lower bad cholesterol levels.

Garlic

Garlic definitely a super food, but then some people just can't get past the smell. Garlic has been used as both food and medicine in many cultures for thousands of years, dating at least as far back as the time that the Giza pyramids were built. In 1858, Louis Pasteur observed garlic's antibacterial activity, and it was used as an antiseptic to prevent gangrene during World War I and World War II.

Garlic given to rats, along with a high protein diet, has been shown to boost testosterone levels. The active ingredient responsible for the testosterone boost in garlic is allicin.

As men get older we naturally lose our testosterone, but, with exercise and a proper diet, it's possible to elevate those levels. Garlic is one weapon in our diet that can help combat the loss of testosterone. Testosterone is very important for muscle, bone mass, fat loss, and a sense of well-being.

Garlic has also been shown to lower cortisol levels. Cortisol causes the breakdown of muscles. Cortisol is released by stress, and is thought to contribute to higher obesity levels in today's society.

I don't use garlic supplements as garlic is something that needs to be fresh in order to obtain all of its health benefits. This is an instance where I believe supplements are a waste of money.

Keep in mind garlic is a blood thinner much like aspirin. Allistatin is an antibiotic found naturally in plants of the Allium group, which includes garlic and onions. It is recognized as being a strong broad-spectrum fungicide and antibiotic against bacteria. The name "allistatin" refers to two very similar recognized compounds, allistatin I and II.

Studies have established that the most active factors in garlic, including allistatin I and allistatin II, are sulphur-containing compounds which are powerful agents against staphylococcus and E. coli, very common bacteria that can cause serious infections and, under certain conditions, can become serious or even fatal. For this reason, Russia and other countries, use garlic routinely and extensively to treat numerous infections and diseases such as whooping cough, flu, and a whole host of infectious diseases of viral and bacterial origin.

Garlic is also claimed to help prevent high blood pressure, cancer and diseases of the heart including atherosclerosis and high cholesterol.

Apart from allistatin, garlic has dozens of other substances (including vitamins, minerals, etc), but allistatin I, II, alliin, allicin, garlicin and ajoine are the strongest antibacterial, antifungal, antiviral, immune-enhancing, and anti-platelet compounds found in large quantities in garlic.

Stick with raw garlic, as much as possible, for its health benefits. Cooking garlic reduces its effectiveness. The older garlic becomes, the less effective it becomes. The best way to prepare garlic is to crush it, and then consume within a few minutes. After an hour most of its health benefits will be gone. Eating parsley may help reduce garlic breath.

Another negative about garlic, of course, is that if you eat too much of it at once it can burn the inside of your stomach pretty good and cause heartburn. Listen to what your body tells you and you can't go wrong. If eating too much garlic is hard on your stomach or gives you a headache for instance, then slow down.

Garlic may be a great food for you to eat on a regular basis based on all the studies out there, but remember everyone is different. Some of us have food allergies and so forth to different kinds of foods so no matter what you eat, pay attention to how you feel afterwards.

Kale

Kale is very high in beta carotene, vitamin K, vitamin C, lutein, zeaxanthin, and calcium. To give you an idea of how many nutrients are in kale, one cup of chopped, boiled kale contains a full day's supply of vitamin A for men or women, and over a 1,000 mcg of vitamin K. The best thing, for those of us on a budget, is, it's cheap.

I do recommend buying organic kale to avoid pesticide exposure, but if it is unaffordable or unavailable, I occasionally will go for the conventional kale that's been pre-washed, which is really inexpensive. Please be aware that kale has been on the top 12 list for pesticide use, so again, go organic as much as possible, if not always, when shopping for kale.

Avoid kale that is soft, brown, or wilted. Get the kale that appears blue green, and dry. Make sure you put it in the fridge and eat it within a few days. If it hasn't been pre-washed, make sure you wash it in cold water.

Kale can be steamed, sautéed, roasted, boiled or eaten raw. Personally, I like to make the leaves into chips by cooking them with coconut oil and salt on a cooking sheet. It tastes great, and makes a very healthy snack.

Women may want to especially take note of this – movie starlets like Gwyneth Paltrow, who played the Black Widow on *Iron Man II*, and Anne Hathaway, who played Catwoman on *The Dark Knight Rises,* both relied on kale as a big part of their diet.

Reported health benefits of kale are reduced risk of some cancers, reduced inflammation, and lower cholesterol. Multiply that by all health benefits of losing fat from switching from processed foods and sugar to kale.

Another other benefit of kale, like all vegetables, is its fiber content, which makes you feel full. The great thing to keep in mind is that good healthy food not only makes you feel full, it provides all the nutrients a person's body needs to thrive. Junk food mostly goes to waste and fat in your body because it's just mostly junk. You can live off a lot less with healthy food verses junk food. Your body isn't going to feel like it's starving all the time like it does with a constant barrage of unsatisfying sugar.

Lentils

Lentils are great primarily because they are not only healthy, but they are cheaper than dirt as well. You can't use expense as an excuse for not eating this health food.

Lentils are very rich in protein, folic acid, and both soluble and insoluble dietary fiber. Lentils are also very high in Vitamin C and the B vitamins, and contain eight of the essential amino acids. They contain many trace minerals, plus iron. Lentils also have a little bit of vitamin K as well.

Several studies indicate that lentils lower the risk of heart disease. Their fiber makes them great for the digestive system, and they can help stabilize blood sugar levels.

Great things sometimes do come cheap!

Mushrooms

Mushrooms are a low-calorie food that can be eaten raw or cooked. Raw dietary mushrooms are a good source of B vitamins, such as riboflavin, niacin and pantothenic acid, and the essential minerals, selenium, copper and potassium. Fat, carbohydrate and calorie content are low. Mushrooms are also a good source of vitamin D.

The biggest plus for mushrooms is that they are low in calories, making them great for losing weight and feeling full at the same time.

A good way to make mushrooms very tasty is to cook them with coconut oil and salt lightly. For added flavor, you can cook them with sliced onions.

Nuts

While nuts do have high fat content and should be consumed in moderation, they are an important healthy snack to add to your diet.

Almonds, for example, are a rich source of vitamin E. They also have dietary fiber, B vitamins, essential minerals and monounsaturated fat, which potentially may lower LDL (bad) cholesterol. Almonds are usually cited as good for weight loss efforts because they help keep you satisfied longer.

In the Bible, nuts are mentioned with the best of fruits in Genesis 43:11: "And their father Israel said unto them, If it must be so now, do this; take of the best fruits in the land in your vessels, and carry down the man a present, a little balm, and a little honey, spices, and myrrh, nuts, and almonds."

Walnuts are said to be good for your brain, and it should be noted that, in fact, walnuts kind of look like a brain as well. Could it be God was trying to tell us something?

Peanuts, though technically part of the legume or bean family, are a significant source of resveratrol, a chemical associated with in studies, but not yet proven to cause, a reduction in risk of cardiovascular disease and cancer.

Peanuts are a source of coenzyme Q10, as are oily fish, beef, soybeans and spinach. CoQ10 is essential for generating the body's energy. The heart, liver, and kidneys have the highest CoQ10 concentrations. Coenzyme Q10 helps to maintain a healthy cardiovascular system. One study showed that by giving rats CoQ10, their life spans were actually lengthened.

The downside to peanuts though, is the fact that some people do have allergies to them, and conventionally grown peanuts are more likely to absorb pesticides due to their soft shells. Nuts, like almonds and walnuts, have strong, hard shells that protect them from pesticides. Peanuts are one of the crops most heavily sprayed with pesticides as well.

Onions

Onions contain chemical compounds believed to have anti-inflammatory effects. They are believed to lower cholesterol, lower risk of cancer, and have antioxidant properties, such as quercetin. Onions are thought to boost your body's natural abilities to protect you from hypertension and osteoporosis.

Studies have shown onions and garlic may provide protection against, esophageal cancer, colon cancer, breast cancer, ovarian cancer, and prostate cancer.

Western Yellow onions have the most flavonoids, eleven times the amount found in Western White, the variety with the lowest flavonoid content. Flavonoids are thought to have anti-cancerous properties.

For all varieties of onions, the more phenols and flavonoids they contain, the more reputed antioxidant and anticancer activity they provide.

Shallots have the most phenols, six times the amount found in Vidalia onion, the variety with the lowest phenolic content. Shallots also have the most antioxidant activity, followed by Western Yellow, Northern Red, Mexico, Empire Sweet, Western White, Peruvian Sweet, Texas 1015, Imperial Valley Sweet, and Vidalia.

The downside to onions of course is the tears they bring to the eyes when cutting them.

Pineapple

Pineapple is a great tasting fruit that provides vitamin C, manganese, fiber, vitamin B6, copper, vitamin B1, and folate. Pineapple is so tasty I can't imagine anyone thinking that junk food could taste better. It is also one of those fruits that are safer from pesticides so you don't necessarily have to buy organic.

Plums

Plums are great to eat right before a workout along with apples, pears, citrus fruit, or berries. Plums can give you a little boost without spiking your insulin too much. Plums contain vitamins C, K, and A. Plums also contain close to three percent of the daily value of potassium. Plums have lots of fiber, making them good for the digestive system. Just like other fruits, plums are good for your eyes.

Make sure you avoid the genetically modified plums as the health effects of GMO plums are currently unknown. A five-digit number beginning with 8 on the produce indicates that it is genetically modified. There have been several studies relating other GM altered foods with possible health issues to the digestive system and even cancer.

Other than that, regular conventional plums are lower on pesticide use, making them a decent option even when the organic variety isn't available.

Salmon

Salmon is considered healthy due to the fish's high protein, high omega-3 fatty acids, and high vitamin D content. You want to avoid farm raised as they will contain more contaminants than the wild caught variety.

Omega-3 comes in three types, alpha-linolenic acid (ALA), docosahexaenoic acid (DHA), and eicosapentaenoic acid (EPA); wild salmon has traditionally been an important source of DHA and EPA, which are important for brain function and structure, among other things. The primary benefit from Omega-3 fatty acids is reducing inflammation throughout the body.

Astaxanthin is a potent antioxidant that stimulates the development of healthy fish nervous systems and enhances the fish's fertility and growth rate. Wild salmon get these carotenoids from eating krill and other tiny shellfish.

The vast majority of Atlantic salmon available on the world market are farmed, up to almost 99%, whereas the majority of Pacific salmon are wild caught, usually greater than 80%. If you look, it should say on the package whether or not it is farm raised or wild caught. Canned salmon in the U.S. is usually wild Pacific catch, though some farmed salmon is available in canned form. In my opinion, the worst fish to get of any kind is going to be fish that is farm raised and comes from China. How many times have you heard of China's products being inferior or even dangerous? I sure wouldn't trust their food enough to eat it on a regular basis.

Unfortunately, mercury is a concern when eating fish. Eating fish is not as healthy of an option as it once was. The smaller the fish caught in the wild, the less mercury it's likely to contain. For this reason, sardines are safer in this regard. It's a shame because salmon is such a great healthy choice otherwise. All things considered, I would still consider salmon a great food. We eat it in our home about twice a week, and we take fish oil supplements to make up the difference in omega-3s. If it weren't for the mercury and contaminants issue, it would be a great food to eat almost every day. Mercury can damage your brain, kidney and lungs.

Spinach

Spinach is high in antioxidants, rich in vitamin A, lutein, vitamin C, vitamin E, vitamin K, magnesium, manganese, folate, betaine, vitamin B2, calcium, potassium, vitamin B6, folic acid, copper, protein, phosphorus, zinc, niacin, selenium, and omega-3 fatty acids.

Eating foods rich in lutein and zeaxanthin can lower your risk of macular degeneration in the eyes, and spinach is especially high in lutein. Foods high in vitamin E may lower risk for dementia and Alzheimer's disease.

Research shows that eating spinach may make you stronger, just not quite as fast as it works for Popeye. The nitrate in spinach is thought to produce nitric oxide, which can increase the flow of oxygen and nutrients to muscles.

One warning about eating too much spinach, if you are prone to kidney stones, spinach contains lots of oxalates, which could increase the risk of kidney stones. To reduce the risk of kidney stones, you might also consider drinking a glass of water with some lemon or lime juice. Limes have virtually no harmful fructose, so they great for adding some taste to your tea or water. Of course just keeping hydrated is very important to avoiding kidney stones as well.

Spinach is near the top of the list of foods with the most pesticide used, so get the organic kind. Fortunately, organic spinach isn't that expensive and isn't usually hard to find either.

Yogurt

Yogurt is nutritionally rich in protein, calcium, riboflavin, vitamin B6, and vitamin B12. It has nutritional benefits beyond those found in milk. People who are moderately lactose-intolerant can consume yogurt without ill effects, because much of the lactose in the milk precursor is converted to lactic acid by the bacterial culture.

Yogurt contains varying amounts of fat. A study conducted in 2005 found that consumption of low-fat yogurt can promote weight loss.

Yogurt is a favorite evening snack for me. I like to add blueberries, walnuts, unsweetened coconut, and a banana. Another favorite I like to mix with yogurt is frozen mango. It tastes like a frozen creamsicle. I get my desert cravings met, and I get lots of vitamins on top of that.

I recommend eating plain, low-fat, organic yogurt. It only cost a little more money. And you'll want to avoid the kinds of yogurt that have added sugar, artificial sweeteners, and so forth.

Yogurt provides probiotics that are actually live microorganisms that are good for our digestive health. These days antibiotics are in our food, as farmers pump it into the livestock to grow bigger animals. The problem is that it may kill the good bacteria in our guts or at least lower the amount of good bacteria we need for our digestion. So yogurt helps us maintain a good healthy balance.

8 ORGANIC FOOD

I talk a lot about organic foods in this book. With some foods it is imperative to buy organic, like apples and spinach, and others, like avocados and pineapples, are much less affected by pesticides.

One thing to look for is the skin of the produce. If it's in a thick skin like an avocado that gets peeled away, it's much less likely to have pesticide contamination.

One huge study into organic food, which was a four-year EU (European Union) funded project called the Quality Low Input Food (QLIF) project, found that organic fruits and vegetables have up to 40 percent more antioxidants than conventionally grown foods and higher levels of minerals like iron and zinc.

Foods to Definitely Buy Organic

These foods are normally very healthy, but it's highly recommended that you buy organic to avoid the conventionally grown versions that rely heavily on pesticides when they are grown.

The site ewg.org has lists that were compiled by the Environmental Working Group (EWG), based on pesticide tests from the U.S. Department of Agriculture and the FDA. You may want to check those out. The higher a food is on the pesticide list, of course, the more you should buy only organic. Produce like apples, celery, strawberries, peaches, spinach, imported nectarines, imported grapes, sweet bell peppers, potatoes, domestic blueberries, lettuce, and kale are all high on the list, with apples topping the chart. I would recommend never eating an apple that was not organic.

Other produce like cilantro, cucumbers, cherries, and pears are high enough on the list to raise some concerns. A few items that you can get away with buying cheaper, conventionally grown due to fewer pesticides being detected are mushrooms, grapefruit, sweet potatoes, watermelon, cabbage, kiwi, domestic cantaloupe, eggplant, mangoes, sweet peas, asparagus, avocado, pineapples, sweet corn, and onions. These are known as being the cleanest conventional foods. Foods like avocados have thick skins that help protect them from the pesticides.

Review the complete clean and dirty produce list from the Environmental Working Group. This is a great list to have handy in the grocery store to help keep your family safe while still keeping costs as low as possible by buying the cheaper conventionally grown produce on the lower pesticide list.

Dirty Dozen Buy These Organic	Clean 15 Lowest in Pesticide
1 Apples	1 Onions
2 Celery	2 Sweet Corn
3 Strawberries	3 Pineapples
4 Peaches	4 Avocado
5 Spinach	5 Asparagus
6 Nectarines - imported	6 Sweet peas
7 Grapes - imported	7 Mangoes
8 Sweet bell peppers	8 Eggplant
9 Potatoes	9 Cantaloupe - domestic
10 Blueberries - domestic	10 Kiwi
11 Lettuce	11 Cabbage
12 Kale/collard greens	12 Watermelon
	13 Sweet potatoes
	14 Grapefruit
	15 Mushrooms

Genetically Modified Foods

Another thing to avoid in fruits and vegetables are genetically modified organism (GMO) foods. There are no real scientific evidence to support the safety of eating GMO foods over a lifetime. Already studies in rats have shown possible health issues with GMO's.

One has to question, for instance, the safety of eating genetically modified corn that is created with the ability to kill the larvae of beetles, such as the corn rootworm. Also of concern is the fact that there are fears that the insects might grow immune to the GMO anyway.

Farmers have been sued for growing some GMO's inadvertently because the GMO seeds have gotten mixed in with their conventional seeds. The GMO companies have actually attacked farmers in court, putting innocent farmers out of business for something completely out of their control.

Bt corn has been equipped with a gene from soil bacteria called Bt (Bacillus thuringiensis), which produces the Bt-toxin, a pesticide that breaks open the stomach of certain insects and kills them. Does that sound like something you want to eat? Concerns are that the GMO corn could interfere with human digestive systems. This is another reason to avoid processed foods, as GMO corn is more than likely used for anything containing high fructose corn syrup. Even animals may be fed the corn from confined animal feeding operations.

Processed foods that should be avoided due to GMO's are products with corn, soy, canola, and any of their derivatives listed as an ingredient, unless it's labeled USDA 100% organic.

While the U.S. does not require GMOs to be labeled, you can still determine whether or not your produce is genetically engineered, organic, or conventional, by looking at its PLU (Price Look Up) code.

For example:

A conventionally grown product carries a 4-digit PLU code (example: conventionally grown banana - 4011)

An organic product carries a 5-digit code, starting with the number 9: (example: organic banana - 94011)

A genetically engineered (GE or GMO) product has a 5-digit code, starting with the number 8: (example: GE banana - 84011)

9 THE MANY HEALTH BENEFITS OF SPICES

Spices aren't just for adding flavor to your meal. They can also add many health benefits as well. Herbs and spices contain antioxidants, minerals and multivitamins and naturally increase your metabolism.

Fingerroot, rosemary, and turmeric are thought to eliminate as much as forty percent of HCAs, which are cancer-causing compounds that are created when meat is barbecued, grilled, broiled or fried. HCA's are thought to cause colorectal, stomach, lung, pancreatic, mammary and prostate cancers. Another way to cut back on HCA's is to cook your food longer and at lower temperatures to avoid burning and creating the HCA's in the first place.

When buying dried spices try to find organic, as regular spices may be irradiated, which may rob some of the spices many healthful benefits.

It is important to keep in mind that when using spices you shouldn't use an excessive amount. Some spices may have side effects if too much is used, and, if you've never had a certain spice before, you may find that you are allergic to it and not even know it. Common sense tells us, of course, that too much of almost anything can be harmful. If you are taking any medications, it's a good idea to consult your doctor or pharmacist before adding new spices to your diet.

Basil

Basil is thought to have anti-bacterial and anti-inflammatory properties. Basil is a very good source of vitamins A, K, C, as well as iron, calcium, potassium, and magnesium.

Cayenne pepper

Cayenne pepper contains vitamins A, E, D, B6, and K, along with fiber and manganese. Of course, cayenne peppers are really hot and spicy due to the capsaicin found in them. There have been many studies on the ability of capsaicin to reduce pain, aid the cardio vascular system, and prevent ulcers, even though they have a bad reputation for causing stomach pain and ulcers. It is thought now that cayenne peppers kill bacteria that causes ulcers.

Capsaicin's peppery heat stimulates secretions that help clear mucus from your stuffed up nose or lungs.

Eating cayenne pepper has a thermogenic effect that may help you lose weight by increasing metabolism.

Cinnamon

Cinnamon has been shown to lower blood sugar, help with digestion, relieve congestion and muscle and joint pain, stimulate circulation. It may help with arthritis, prevent urinary tract infections, tooth decay, and gum disease. It can kill E. coli and other bacteria. Cinnamon is a good source of calcium, manganese, and fiber.

On the downside, too much cinnamon has been known to be bad for the liver. People with liver trouble may want to stay away from cinnamon, as well as those taking certain medications, like acetaminophen, which are tough on the liver.

Cinnamon is mentioned in the Bible in Exodus 30:23, as one of the component parts of the holy anointing oil, Proverbs 7:17, Song of Solomon 4:14, and Revelation 18:13. One of its main uses in the Bible days was as a perfume.

Proverbs 7:17
I have perfumed my bed with myrrh, aloes, and cinnamon.

Cloves

Cloves are a good source of manganese, omega-3 fatty acids, vitamin K, dietary fiber, vitamin C, calcium and magnesium. Cloves are known for their anti-inflammatory, anti-bacterial, and antioxidant properties. They also help with respiratory problems, like asthma and bronchitis, and aid in relief of muscle pain. They are known as well for eliminating intestinal parasites, fungi, and bacteria. They may even help with mental focus. Too much clove oil can have side effects like increased bleeding and lowered blood sugar. People with allergies to clove may show signs of a rash, itching or shortness of breath.

Ginger

Ginger is known for its ability to help relieve nausea and for eliminating intestinal gas. Like many other spices, it has anti-inflammatory properties and antioxidants. Ginger is said to relieve dizziness, boost the immune system, protect against bacteria, encourage bile flow, and help your cardiovascular system. One study indicated that ginger could be more effective at treating sea sickness than Dramamine.

Studies have been done that indicate that ginger may be helpful for arthritis suffers. Ginger contains very powerful anti-inflammatory compounds called gingerols.

One study even showed promise that ginger could slow growth of colorectal cancer cells. Another showed that ginger actually killed ovarian cancer cells.

To get the best results from ginger, buy the fresh root instead of the dried kind on the spice racks. Make sure the ginger is firm, smooth, and free of mold before purchasing. To prepare, remove the skin from fresh, mature ginger with a paring knife. It can then be sliced, minced or julienned. The longer ginger is cooked the less pungent it tastes.

Don't overdo ginger, though, as quantities in excess of two grams of ginger per kilogram of body weight can cause an acute overdose, which can lead to a state of over-stimulation of the central nervous system called ginger intoxication or the "ginger jitters". It's always a good idea to remember even too much of a good thing can be bad for you.

Although it is generally considered to be safe, powdered ginger may cause heartburn, bloating, gas, belching and nausea. Ginger may also cause adverse effects in people suffering from gallstones because it promotes the production of bile. Those who have had ulcers, inflammatory bowel disease or blocked intestines may have a bad reaction to large quantities of fresh ginger.

Oregano

Oregano, used primarily in Mediterranean and Mexican dishes, contains vitamin K, manganese, iron, fiber, calcium, and vitamin E. Oregano contains the oils thymol and carvacrol, which are known to slow down the growth of bacteria. Oregano contains many phytonutrients, like thymol and rosmarinic acid, that act as powerful antioxidants. Here's an amazing fact: oregano has demonstrated 42 times more antioxidant activity than apples, 30 times more than potatoes, 12 times more than oranges, and 4 times more than blueberries, on a per gram weight basis.

When shopping for oregano, buy the fresh kind that is vibrant green in color and has firm stems. Oregano should be added toward the end when cooking, so it does not lose its flavor.

Peppermint

Fresh peppermint has vitamin A, manganese, and vitamin C. Peppermint has been shown to help with stomach problems like irritable bowel syndrome and other digestion problems. Animal studies have shown peppermint to stop pancreatic, mammary, and liver tumors from growing. Peppermint helps with asthma through a substance it contains called rosmarinic acid, which opens up airways for better breathing.

Too much peppermint oil can cause issues related to slower heartbeat, rapid breathing, depression, or even unconsciousness, as well as other issues.

Thyme

Thyme contains vitamin K, iron, manganese, calcium, fiber, and tryptophan. Tryptophan may help with appetite regulation, better sleep, and mood. Tryptophan is also found in chicken, soybeans, tuna, turkey, salmon, lamb, halibut, shrimp, and cod.

But back to thyme itself, which may be helpful in dealing with chest congestion issues. In fact, it has a long history of being used for that purpose. Thyme has also found to be potentially beneficial to brain, kidney, and heart cell membranes.

Thyme has a reputation for killing bacteria dead. It's known to combat Staphalococcus aureus, Bacillus subtilis, Escherichia coli and Shigella sonnei.

Turmeric

Lots of research is going on right now on the health benefits of turmeric. Turmeric is grown in India and other tropical regions of Asia. It looks like an orange-yellow powder. Turmeric is thought to improve digestion, support a healthy liver, fight cancer, inflammation, and arthritis.

10 WEIGHT TRAINING

Weight training is one of the best ways to get into shape, just ahead of cardio. Weight training builds muscle, which gives you a higher resting metabolism. That means the more muscle you have, the more fat you burn, even when you aren't exercising at that moment. Cardio burns fat primarily only while you are doing the exercise. Another great thing about weight training is that it helps us maintain bone density as we grow older, making weight training especially important for women.

With weight training, the idea is to keep your muscles guessing. For beginners, just doing any sort of workout will shock the muscles into gains. After a person has been lifting for a good while, it is necessary to modify workout routines more frequently to continue to see muscle growth. The more the muscles get used to a workout, the less likely they are to respond with positive growth.

Personally, I love to change out my routine as much as possible every week. Even if I do bench press every chest day, I may do it slightly different from week to week. For example, I might drop the weight slowly, and pause on my chest before driving it quickly upward again. The next week, I might bring the weight down and up as fast as I can, or go down slow and up fast, or do something different every set. Once muscles get used to a certain routine they do not respond with gains anymore.

Never stretch before a workout. Do your stretches after you're done with the workout. Studies now have shown that a person is more likely to get injured or tear a muscle if they stretch before a workout, as it may actually temporarily weaken the muscle. It is still a good idea to stretch at the end of the workout to keep yourself flexible and to keep your muscles from being as sore for the next day or so. Always do some light warm-up exercises before a workout to avoid injury. Gradually increase the weight on each exercise, at least until you've gotten the muscle group you are working that day sufficiently warm and pumped with blood.

Weight Training For Fat Loss

I have found that I lose the most fat with high intensity weight training exercises.

There are several ways to increase the intensity of a workout. You could do split routines, similar to what Arnold Schwarzenegger performed back in his body building competition days. Arnold would do bench press for example and without more than a minute or so rest he would go straight to chin-ups.

Really, the set pattern of your workout depends on your own personal fitness level and how bad you want to lose fat and build muscle. But to lose fat, I find the less I take in rest between sets, and the harder I push it on the weights the more I lose. Everyone is different, so play around with different workouts and see what gives you the most results. Again, if you are just starting out, it doesn't take much to see results, so take it slow at first and build up.

Beginners, and those of us that have been at it a while, you got to eat right or it doesn't matter how much you work out in terms of weight loss. Sure, you burn calories and you'd be thinner than if you sat on the couch, but if you have a junk food diet, the weight will always catch up to you.

Some ideas to help you once you realize your workout routines aren't cutting it anymore are to, as I've said, ramp up the intensity, cut the rests in between sets, and go to muscle failure on the last couple of sets you do. Basically, you want to push your body hard enough that it has to sink way down deep on those fat reserves. Be careful though, it's a fine line between hitting it just right and over training, which I can tell you is really hard on the old nervous system. So don't do intense workouts for too long a duration. Overtraining can make you sick, and if you miss your workout the next day you might lose ground. So don't work out longer than what you can recover from by your next scheduled workout.

Another thing you can do to up the intensity level if you hit a plateau is to mix cardio with the weight training. Do some jump rope, then do your weight lifting set, or maybe use a punching bag, or jump as high as you can 10 to 20 times and then go back to the weights. Give yourself a minute of rest between each set, or at least 30 seconds depending upon your own personal conditioning. Beginners may need a lot more rest between sets.

Weight Training for Strength

Weight training for strength is more about getting the most weight lifted during the shortest amount of reps. When I'm doing a strength training cycle, I'll take my time and maybe yack about nothing to people in the gym between sets because I'm wanting to get really rested between sets. It's not a bad idea though to throw in a few high rep exercises toward the end to get the blood flowing good. Also, warm up really well. You don't want to tire yourself out, but at the same time you need blood flowing to the muscle groups you are about to work. It's very easy when you are going for the heavy weight to pull a muscle which really can set you back a long way. So take the time to warm up. You'll lift heavier anyway, if your muscles are warm and pumped up with blood, than if you just jump into a workout cold.

My personal training is usually more about an all-around fitness level. I want to be able to run, jump, and be as strong as possible at the same time. Weight training helps with these goals, but one should be careful not to avoid cardio. Guys who don't focus on the cardio and some level of flexibility training tend to get injured more. Balance is key for long term success.

I've been weight training for well over 25 years now, even though a lot of those years I could have done a lot better if I would have avoided the health pitfalls I'm warning you about in this book. I've seen guys work out for years and are still going strong, and at the same time I've seen a few guys who, while they are still at it, do have some regrets on how their training could have gone better. The bottom line is it's better to train for longevity than to try to be the Hulk in a year. Smart body builders warm up and they lift heavy weights, but in perfect form. They also know how to use lighter weights to get excellent results.

Working out with your buds is great for motivation, but it can be a double edged sword, if you pull muscles and wind up in the hospital trying to impress the guys at the gym. The idea is to build up your body and not destroy it. So work out with intensity, yes, and with as much as you can put into it, but temper that enthusiasm by doing the exercises with correct form.

Again, it's important to switch things around from time to time so your body doesn't get used to one type of workout, and thus end your muscle growth.

Body Building Techniques

The difference between strength training and body building comes down to the output desired. A body builder wants to put the focus on the muscles. A strength trainer or power lifter only cares about how much weight they lift. Those goals may seem to go hand in hand, and they do to a certain point, but the body builder will take curls, for example, and do the strictest form necessary to tax the bicep muscle and nothing else, whereas the strength trainer is more focused on moving the weight from point A to point B.

That's not to say body builders don't use extremely heavy weights sometimes, but they tend to use lighter weights a lot more often than power lifters. If the power lifter misses a few muscles in training he or she may not care as long as it doesn't interfere with how much weight they lift, but the body builder is concerned with getting every muscle he or she needs worked to get the look they are trying to achieve. It is appearance verses functionality, but a person will benefit physically from either approach.

Abs

No matter what exercise you do, the abs become engaged to some degree. Sit-ups, some say, are actually bad on the back, and have been replaced by the crunch to some extent. There are a variety of abs specific exercises one can employ to build up abs muscles, via gym equipment or just working out at home. If you are using weight, it is a good idea to choose a weight that allows you to do at least 25 reps or more. You don't want the muscles in your stomach area to become too thick or it will cause your stomach to stick out, which is not the desired effect. By doing high reps you can strengthen the abs without creating a bulky look.

The key to great abs ultimately lies in your diet. No matter how much you work the abs, if you have too much fat it will just cover up the muscle. Spot training doesn't work either. A thousand sit-ups burns some calories, but a couple of cokes a day will just add those calories right back on. So if you are serious about having great abs, ditch the ice cream, sodas, chips, cookies, and basically anything with added sugar or processed junk food. Eat real food, and drink water, tea, or something without sugar or artificial sweeteners, and you are on your way to having great abs.

Planks are a great isometric exercise for the abs and your entire core. To do a front plank, place your elbows on the ground directly beneath your shoulders and hold your body up on your forearms and toes. It's similar to a push-up, but you hold your position on the elbows instead of pushing up and down.

Doing crunches on a stability ball is another great way to work your abs. Just lie down on an inflated stability ball and crunch forward with your feet planted firmly on the ground. This is easy to do while you watch TV and really burns your abs.

Curls

For the body builder, the best way to get the most results in arm training is to use light enough weights to allow a full contraction of the muscle. The arms should be extended all the way down and then all the way back up again. The weight should be enough that within 20 reps you reach the point of exhaustion. Again, the primary focus is contracting the bicep muscle, so the entire focus must be on that muscle as one does the exercise.

Bench Press

The bench press focuses on the chest, shoulders, and triceps. While body builders tend to use less weight for curls, they tend to go much heavier with the bench press. Still, the focus is putting the emphasis on the muscle and not just moving the weight. The bench press is a favorite of power lifters as well, but the focus is primarily on strength.

Weak triceps can reduce the amount of weight you can lift on the bench press. So it is a good idea to do at least one to two other exercises for your triceps every week.

It's always a good idea to have a spotter when doing bench press. It's almost impossible to get the most out of the bench press without one. Not only does not having a spotter prevent you from ever reaching muscle failure, if you do reach muscle failure, getting the bar off of your chest can be a massive pain, opening up a good chance for injury.

Pull-ups

The pull-up is the best exercise for building strength and shaping your back. Most gyms have a pull-up bar you can use for this exercise. To perform this exercise, you should grasp the bar and pull yourself up to chin level. If you are not strong enough to do a pull-up on your own, you can have someone spot you by standing behind you and holding your feet as you pull yourself up. Advanced body builders may use belts to attach additional weight in order to lift more weight in fewer reps and shape an overall larger back.

Squats

The basic squat with a loaded barbell on a lifter's back is a great full body exercise. It primarily works the muscles of the thighs, hamstrings, buttocks, quads, and hips, but also isometrically works the core, upper back and shoulders.

Performing squats an actually increase bench press strength. I find it most beneficial to space out the day I do squats and the day I do bench press each week. This allows for recuperation time so I can lift heavier weight and perform more reps with less risk of injury, since both exercises use the same muscle groups to some extent.

Some argue that you should always wear a protective weight lifting belt to protect your back, but others believe that wearing a belt prevents strengthening of the core. One recent study, however, showed that wearing a belt actually engaged the abdominal muscles more than not wearing a belt.

111

The Body Builder Diet

For those focused on building a body builder physique, what you eat is just as important as weight lifting technique. Primarily, think protein via lean meat, like chicken breasts. As I said before, the best chicken breasts to get are the organic variety that contain no antibiotics.

Eggs are key. Eggs went from the unhealthy list back to the healthy list due to the cholesterol in the egg yolk. Now studies are showing that cholesterol is healthy for us, and eggs give us another source of good quality protein for muscle building.

Testosterone, of course, is essential to building muscle. And what is the natural healthy way to increase testosterone? Avoid processed foods like the plague! Chemicals in canned goods and other processed foods can actually mess with your hormones and lower your testosterone.

Try adding crushed garlic to your food. Garlic supplementation in rats, along with a high protein diet, has been shown to boost testosterone levels, but don't bother with supplements. Stick with the real thing. The active ingredient responsible for the testosterone boost in garlic is allicin. It's most beneficial within a few minutes of being crushed. Garlic is also a blood thinner. It helps fight inflammation. The only negative, besides the smell, is the heartburn it might cause. Make sure you mix it well with your food and try small amounts at first to make sure you can stomach it.

Protein shakes are great when you don't have much time. The most important time to get protein into your body is before and after a workout. Consuming protein after a workout is especially important because your muscles are primed and ready to take in protein and other nutrients.

You should eat healthy fats like that found in salmon and avocados, but never within a few hours before or after a workout. Your body is less efficient in using fat during and directly after a workout. Eating fat during this time can actually make you a little sick too.

Steroids

I probably don't even have to mention the dangers of steroid use. Steroids may bring amazing short term benefits, but they are not worth it in the long haul. Consider professional wrestlers, the sport reported to have the highest use of steroids, and then look at how many professional wrestlers die early deaths.

Probably one of the most common users of steroids in America today are the young high school athletes who want desperately to win at their sport and perhaps get a college scholarship or even prepare for a professional career. Adults need to pay particular attention to the warning signs of steroid use, like mood swings and rapid muscle gain in a very short period of time.

Having said that, some do estimate that fifty percent of steroid users aren't even athletes. They are just people trying to look better.

Lyle Alzado, who won a championship in Super Bowl XVIII as a player with the Los Angeles Raiders, blamed steroids for his battle with brain cancer that eventually took his life at the age of 43.

Steve Michalik won a number of body building titles including the 1971 AAU Mr. USA, the Mr. America in 1972, and the NABBA Mr. Universe in 1975, as well as 22 other titles including the 1971 AAU Mr. Apollo and the Most Muscular Man in the USA. Michalik claimed he used steroids for ten years. His use first began in preparation for the 1975 Mr. Universe competition.

According to Michalik, he suffered many serious health problems due to his steroid use. It started with him passing blood in his urine; a sign of the multiple liver tumors doctors later discovered. After recovering from these bouts with cancer, Michalik suffered a heart attack, followed by a stroke. From then on, he was against the use of steroids. Michalik died on May 24, 2012. He was 63.

Common issues with steroids in men are breast swelling, shrinking of testicles, and bad acne. In women, often there is a permanent deepening of the voice, male pattern baldness, facial hair, and shrinking of the breasts.

Doctors believe steroids cause tumors on the liver and the kidneys. Steroids are thought to increase the risk of heart attack and stroke by lowering the good cholesterol in the body. This, in turn, causes plaque buildup in the arteries. Some doctors suggest the buildup in thirty year old steroid abusers to be similar to that of those in their seventies.

The temptation to be the best in athletics or to have the best body is great for some, but like all things that are too good to be true, that is especially true for steroids. Having a great physique is very doable through weight training and a proper diet, and the benefits can improve the length and quality of life. Steroid use produces short term results, but the consequences are not worth it. The whole point of physical fitness shouldn't be about one moment or a couple of years of glory, but about helping make people healthier throughout their lives. Who cares if you can bench more than Superman if you're dead in ten years. You can't bench anything if you're dead. Just as the Bible says - pride does go before destruction. Wisdom demands that we never put our long term health below short term gains for the sake of impressing others.

Dealing with Injuries

Injuries are a part of exercising unfortunately. Let's face it, especially as we get a little older, a person can get hurt opening a bathroom stall at church. An injury can happen any time any place, even when we aren't working out, so please don't use the excuse of avoiding injuries to not workout. Working out is still a lot safer than sitting on a couch. In fact, the other day I read some poor kid actually died while playing a video game for several hours straight. Evidence mounts more every week as to the dangers of a sedentary lifestyle. I would much rather deal with a pulled muscle occasionally than having to stay in the hospital while my chest is ripped open for heart surgery. So, if working out and getting a few muscle strains means avoiding major surgery, count me in.

The trick is to avoid injuries as much as possible, and if you do get an injury, allow yourself some recuperation time to get it healed as quickly as possible so you can get back into the game. If you get hurt, sometimes you have to take a couple weeks off and revaluate where you are. Going crazy with the weights after you've pulled a muscle could just worsen the injury until you wind up having to have surgery, like rotator cuff shoulder surgery. Avoiding hospital stays is the name of the game, after all, so make sure you put your thinking cap on when it comes to working out safely.

The Dangers of Showing Off

Don't let pride get in the way of working out safely, especially when it comes to weightlifting. It is a good idea to work out with other people if it motivates you, but don't let your pride push you to lift as much weight as people twice your size or people that have been working out twice as long as you have. The idea is to gradually increase your reps and/or weight from week to week. If you manage to impress your friends this week, that's great, but what about next week when you can't lift a spoon to feed yourself without screaming in pain? Always think long term. Hey, even the biggest guys in the gym get taken down from an injury. So what if a guy can bench 350 pounds once in his life, but now he can't even do a pushup.

The idea is to be healthy for as long as possible. If you are a person that thinks competitively, like I do, just consider – the game of life is won by longevity. I want to be the strongest 40 year old I can be, the strongest 50 year old, 60 year old, 70 year old, and Lord willing, on and on as long as possible. When you get down to it, the competition is with yourself, but it's nice to know you're competitive with guys half your age while your peers are wasting away on the couch.

I think in the long term a person will find the most success in their fitness goals by working out for themselves. I know a guy at our gym, who is honestly a pretty big guy, who complained to me once about the injuries he suffered from while trying to impress the other fellows in the gym. He said to me that it's not worth it when you're in a hospital bed wondering where are all the guys I was trying to impress. This is an especially important lesson for teenagers. Don't worry about impressing people. Impress yourself in the gym, and be patient. You've got plenty of time to build up your body. Fitness is not a sprint. It's a marathon.

I remember seeing a group of teens come into the gym one day doing heavy squats. These guys were just asking to be put into wheelchairs. They were at least helping each other out, but they were throwing around at least 315 pounds on their backs, and I bet they didn't weigh more than a 150 pounds apiece. It wasn't that the weight was beyond reason, but to do that much weight without the proper form can be dangerous. Every one of those kids was wobbling around with the weight, about to drop it, and then one actually did. It's a miracle he didn't throw his back out permanently. The owner of the gym had offered to teach them proper form, but the kids refused. Some teens have been blessed with all knowledge at birth, I guess. In reality, of course, it's just being too proud to learn from more experienced weight lifters, and that kind of pride can kill a person.

Working out and eating right can give you years of energy and vitality, but its benefits eventually stop once you stop taking part. That's why dealing with injuries is so important. The best athlete in the world can die an early death once they retire and stop training and eating right. In fact, I think a lot of athletes make the mistake of giving up on working out once they retire. They've made their money and met their goals, but they've forgotten the most important goal of all, and that's a long healthy active life.

God has given us a great gift in that we don't necessarily have to be rich to have a healthy life. He's given us some say so on our health. We are stewards of our bodies. It's our God given responsibility to take care of ourselves. Nobody, not the government, or even your own mother, can do push-ups and pull-ups for you. There are no magic pills that can take the place of good old exercise and healthy food.

Sure, it helps to have money for the best food and best doctors, but if a person doesn't eat the right foods and use the body God gave them, all the money in the world isn't going to add years to their lives.

Concentration

Take each set seriously, as if this set was the one that could tear a muscle. Concentrating before each set makes a huge difference in avoiding injuries. It's always when you are not paying attention, and just going through the motions, that an injury occurs. I've hurt myself more times doing weight that I should have been able to easily than when I was lifting weight that was so heavy it scared me. A healthy fear makes a man or woman focus on lifting that weight and concentrate on the lift. When every muscle is ready, and your mind is sharp you, are in a much safer territory than when you think you've got it no problem. Of course, I'm not saying it's best to lift crazy heavy weight all the time. On the contrary, you should only lift weight you know you can lift safely. You can add weight slowly from week to week, but always take the weight seriously, even on the low weights you use for the warm-up. Always make sure you have the correct form for the exercise you are performing.

Warm Up

Always, always, always warm-up before lifting anything heavy or running full speed. Without getting blood into the muscle first you are just asking to get injured.

Stretching

Don't do static stretching before weightlifting. Studies show it weakens the muscle and could lead to an injury. Warm up before a workout and save the stretching for the end of the workout.

Taking Care of an Injury

Here are some tips that have helped me that I think could be helpful to you, short of going to a doctor. Remember, I'm not advising anyone to avoid seeing a doctor in the event of an injury. These are just some good tips and information from my personal experiences and research. When in doubt, by all means see your doctor.

Injuries heal the fastest when blood is circulating in the body as close to the injured muscle as possible. So, after a short rest period, it's a good idea to try to do some easy exercises that pump blood into the injured area. In fact, if you hurt your leg for instance, and can do so with no pain, it's usually a good idea to keep exercising other body parts. Once your torn muscle has started to heal, carefully work closer to that target area. But If you feel pain, stop.

In general, one heals faster by moving and doing something rather than sitting all day. Try some easy walking. Do anything to keep the body moving. Every injury is different, but for the most part careful movement and good nutrition are key to healing faster. Back pain, especially, does much better with movement verses just lying around, which can actually make back pain worse. In the old days, doctors actually advised patients to lay in bed for a back pain, not realizing it only made things worse.

I've had a few very bad back injuries in my time. I once lost control of light weight during squats. My back lunged forward and the weight jerked backwards. At first, I continued to work out, which was a mistake. Always call it a day when you injure yourself during a workout. Give yourself a chance to determine the extent of your injury. Sometimes an injury gets worse after a night's sleep, and, if you keep working out the day of the injury, you will only make it worse. The next day after my squat incident I could barely get out of bed. I literally had to roll around in the bed in agony for several minutes before I could stand. The pain was almost unbearable, but by moving around the pain would subside, for the most part, by the afternoon, only to come back with a vengeance in the morning. Today, I don't have much trouble with my back, except, perhaps, for an occasional flare up. I find that drinking water and keeping hydrated helps me with the occasional back ache.

I take supplements that help fight inflammation, like fish oil, astaxanthin, and reservatrol. You want to keep the inflammation down to keep the pain down. Avoid sugar at all costs after an injury. Sugar will just cause your body to inflame more. If you are nursing an injury, it is probably a good idea to skip any cheat meals you have planned. Try eating more wild caught salmon than usual. There is no better source for fish oil than real fish, and no better fish than salmon.

If you can stand it, garlic is a great natural way to alleviate inflammation and help with healing injuries. It basically thins your blood the same way aspirin and fish oil do. It also gives you a natural testosterone boost.

Shoulder Injuries and Maintenance

This past year I've struggled with a rotator cuff injury in my shoulder. My right shoulder literally popped when I moved it. At times I was unable to even do a proper set of bench press due to the pain it caused. In many cases, surgery is necessary to repair shoulder injuries. Coincidentally, two of my favorite childhood movie actors, Arnold Schwarzenegger and Sylvester Stallone, were shown side by side in a photo, in a hospital, both getting work done on their shoulders. Interestingly enough, one famous shoulder exercise named after Arnold Schwarzenegger, the Arnold Press, is reputed to cause shoulder problems.

By incorporating shoulder maintenance exercises, utilizing very light weight, I've been able to, once again, see my bench press moving forward instead of backwards. As I write this, I'm now 41 years of age, and at my age I can attest that shoulder injuries do take quite a while to heal. Doing smaller exercises, that focus on the muscles surrounding the ball joint of the shoulder, helps to support and stabilize the shoulder, preventing injury, and, in my case, has helped me recover from a shoulder injury. I'm also a firm believer that healing is in the blood. The more blood you can get to an injury without aggravating the injury, the quicker recovery will happen.

Be careful using dumbbells instead of a barbell for bench press. If you use heavy weights, you can injure your shoulder worse due to the lack of control. Having to throw up the dumbbells to get them in position can rip your shoulder muscle worse.

Below are some of the exercises that have worked for me. The first one, I believe, has done the most good for me personally. If you feel pain, you should go even lighter if you are using weights, or use only your body weight. You should be able to do the movements without any sort of pain whatsoever.

Shoulder Maintenance Exercises

1.   Side shoulder rotation exercise – Lay on the side. Use a very light weight, or no weight at all. Bend the elbow at a 90 degree angle. Then rotate arm up and down from the floor to just a little above shoulder height doing as many reps as is comfortable. My object is to get the shoulder to feel a little burn without pulling or causing any pain; the goal being to circulate blood flow into the shoulder area.

2.   Arm circles – No weights. Hold arms straight out to the sides at shoulder height. Rotate slowly, first in one direction, then the other. You should feel a healthy burning, but not any sharp pains.

3.   Side to side – With arms straight out to the sides, move them straight up and down to your side and back up again slowly. This would be the

same arm motion as a jumping jack, without the jumping, and doing it slowly.

4.   Wall shoulder press – Hold your back and arms against the wall. Stand up straight and press hands up as if holding weights. Working on posture here, so use no weights.

5.   Shoulder push-up – Get into push-up position, but instead of going all the way up and down I push up and down with my shoulders only. Actually, I've done this exercise standing up pushing against a wall, as well, just to get blood flowing to the shoulder area.

Shoulder Exercises to Avoid

1.   The Arnold Press, some say, can lead to injury of the rotator cuff.
2.   Behind the neck press also may lead to a shoulder injury.
3.   Behind the neck lat pull downs can cause rotator cuff injury.

Get to Blood to an Injury

The Bible tells us that the life of the flesh is in the blood. It took centuries before modern doctors caught on to the fact that people would do better if blood was added to a body, rather than taking it out, like what was done in George Washington's day.

> Leviticus 17:11
> For the life of the flesh is in the blood: and I have given it to you upon the altar to make an atonement for your souls: for it is the blood that maketh an atonement for the soul.

Every time I've ever gotten any injury, I've focused on pumping that area up with light weight exercises with a great deal of success. I don't know how many times I've been able to come back from an injury by using that method. Sometimes it works more quickly than others. Areas like the shoulder, where less blood flows, take longer to heal.

The trick is to exercise the area in a way that doesn't aggravate it further, or cause any further damage, and yet can pump blood into that area. It doesn't take much to get a muscle pumped sometimes.

Tendon Injuries

Tendons are small, strong, thick bands of connective tissue that connect the muscle to the bone. They can be injured through a sudden acute tear during the lifting of a heavy weight, or through gradual chronic wear and tear. Working through the pain of a tendon injury can make it worse. When a tendon is injured, the power of your muscles during an exercise cannot be fully converted into the desired movement, thus, essentially preventing the person from lifting as much with the same amount of force. Surgery is the only option for complete tendon ruptures in order to ever resume effective muscle training again. The tendon may be stitched back together, replaced, or screwed back into position. Partial tendon tears can heal on their own given enough time. Many weightlifters push through the pain and keep training. They use pain killers, anti-inflammatories, or cortisone shots, but these may hurt the tendon's recovery in the long run by robbing the tendon of its strength.

Muscle injuries tend to heal much faster than tendon injuries due to the fact that muscles receive much more blood than tendons. In general, lifting weights can increase tendon strength, but tendons get stronger at a much slower rate than muscles because of the greater blood flow into muscles. This is a good reason for newcomers to weight training to take it slow and build up. This allows their tendon strength to catch up with their muscle strength and hopefully prevent a tendons issue.

If you are worried about injuring your tendons, then you should avoid fast negative moves. That's when there is the most pressure on the tendons. Lower the weight more slowly to prevent strain on tendons.

And if you need another reason to avoid sugar – it can make your tendons more brittle.

Here's an interesting fact about tendon strength: A tendon that is about half an inch thick can support a weight of over 1000 pounds.

Avoid Aspirin for Muscle Pain

According to some doctors, aspirin may have the unfortunate side effect of breaking down muscle. This is just the opposite of what you want to happen when you are trying to build muscle.

Not to get sidetracked, but, from time to time, doctors and health practitioners will disagree on some areas of health and fitness. Many doctors swear by the aspirin a day for heart health, but not all doctors agree with that plan. Taking a daily aspirin for heart health isn't something you should do lightly. Talk to your doctor, of course, but the evidence suggests that it's not something someone that is already in good health should necessarily do.

Personally, I would rather depend more on fish oil supplements and garlic for a healthy heart and blood flow. Calcium supplements should be avoided because they may clog arteries, unlike calcium found in food that lowers the possibility of a heart attack.

I know from my own personal experience than when I was taking the recommended aspirin a day, I pulled muscles on a regular basis, including one very painful chest muscle strain. In my case, the problem seemed to correct itself once I stopped taking aspirin.

Of course, everyone is likely aware of the stomach ulcer problem associated with aspirin.

A lot of professional athletes now refuse to take anti-inflammatory drugs for fear of possible kidney problems.

Another popular pain medication, ibuprofen, has caused me injuries as well. I can just about mark it down that if I take an anti-inflammatory medication I will likely to pull a muscle almost every time.

The same goes for Benadryl, an allergy medication, which drains muscles of fluid, leading to injury.

You want to avoid acetaminophen, found in medicines like Tylenol, because they are terrible on the liver. Some reports indicate that acetaminophen is the most common cause of liver damage.

I'm not saying that there isn't a time and a place for anti-inflammatory medication, but take them cautiously, rather than for every occasional ache and pain.

NSAIDs, or Nonsteroidal anti-inflammatory drugs, are generally associated by the medical community with a doubled risk of symptomatic heart failure in patients without a history of cardiac disease. These include ibuprofen and naproxen. NSAIDs are not recommended by doctors during pregnancy, particularly during the third trimester.

One thing I've been able to do by exercising on a consistent basis is see things for myself. I've seen how well anti-inflammatory supplements like fish oil work in controlling aches and pains and in helping me actually heal faster. I've also noticed how well the spice turmeric works to lower inflammation in the body. Everything that works to lower inflammation naturally in the body also helps to lower risk of heart attack without the side effects.

Injuries are going to come in life whether you work out or not. If you don't get hurt lifting weights or running, eventually you'll find yourself getting hurt just bending over to pick up a pencil. The body just deteriorates the less we use it. Sitting still is not good for the body. As more and more studies suggest, the more we sit, the greater chance we have of a heart attack. No matter where you are in life, most likely you can do something. If you can't sprint, then jog, if you can't jog then walk, if you can't walk then crawl, pick up weights, stand up more often, stretch, rotate your neck, anything at all. If you can move it then do it. You'll be better off for it.

The more you can move, the more circulation your body has, and, as I've mentioned before, as the Bible says, "the life is in the blood". You have to get the blood flowing to be as healthy as you can be.

Tips for Back Pain

Occasionally, I have over trained in the gym and wound up pulling my back out doing squats. I've found a few things that help me heal faster and make life more bearable. The first thing is, you may experience your worst back pain in the morning when getting out of bed. I have found that moving around on the bed for a minute before I get up can make a big difference. I'm talking about days when getting out of bed hurts like a rattlesnake bite. Slowly getting the blood flowing into the back area, by moving my legs around, and maybe doing some small ab related movements, seems to help me get out of bed during the times I've had a bad back injury. The second thing you should do is drink some water as soon as you get up. Being dehydrated always makes back pain worse. Obviously, you want to avoid any sugar at all, even from fruit, during a recovery from a painful injury. I've found that anti-inflammatory supplements like fish oil, resveratrol, vitamin D, and astaxanthin make a big difference, as well, along with eating salmon, and adding garlic to my food. Of course, when in doubt, don't be afraid to see a doctor, but the above mentioned items have helped me through some pretty bad back pain in the past.

As I've mentioned, back injuries tend to heal faster and feel much better when you move around as opposed to sitting still all day. Lying in bed can make a back ache worse instead of better.

The Ultimate Safe Workout Plan

For the average person whose main goal is health and longevity, the best way to work out and avoid injuries is to use light weights and do more reps, or slow the movement down. Slowing down the movement makes even the lightest of weights feel heavy after a few reps. Unless you are competing as a power lifter, light weights will work just fine. Many professional body builders use light weights for exercises like bicep training, where the goal is to target the bicep and avoid throwing the weights up. Throwing weights up during curling can cause a back injury. By using a weight you can safely lower all the way down and lift back up again several times, you can really pump up the muscle without pulling or tearing anything.

Testosterone

Testosterone is made from cholesterol, and one of its primary functions is to build muscle, but it also gives men the drive to compete and to succeed. Women also have testosterone, but it's seven times less than the amount found in men. Testosterone is also very important in terms of confidence, sense of well-being, bone mass, and fat loss.

From the womb fetuses are exposed to testosterone. Studies show that testosterone controls the preferences men make, even as young boys. Boys naturally choose toy trucks for instance. In one study with monkeys, even boy monkeys chose toy trucks over dolls, whereas the female monkeys chose the dolls. This shows that nature, not training determines the importance men place on subjects like muscle cars, sports, and hunting over pursuing more feminine interests like hair styles and makeup.

One fascinating study showed that men playing sports showed increases in testosterone while playing a sports game. While both teams showed increases in testosterone by mid game, the winning team's testosterone levels were higher than those of the losing team. Further, the losing team's testosterone levels decreased, but were still higher than at the beginning of the game. Thus, one might conclude that the best way to increase testosterone for men naturally is to get involved in a sport. Even men who were just watching the game in question showed some signs of increased testosterone.

Apparently, we men have testosterone in more abundance in times that we need it the most. The greater the challenge physically or competitively, the greater surge of testosterone a man can experience.

Don't let the food you eat reduce your testosterone. Chemicals in processed foods have been found to decrease testosterone. So eat organic and keep your testosterone levels higher. Also avoid alcohol, which can lower testosterone.

Garlic is one food that can naturally increase testosterone. The active ingredient responsible for the testosterone boost in garlic is allicin. Find more about garlic in Chapter 7.

Anything you can do to increase your testosterone levels naturally can help you reap the health benefits of testosterone without side effects.

11 STRESS MANAGEMENT

Manage Your Money Wisely

I know you're asking, "What does money management have to do with being healthy?" However, it does play a part in our health. It's not necessary to be filthy rich, but being in debt can cause a lot of stress and harm to your body over time, especially if the debt that has become unmanageable.

It's much healthier and easier on the body to not have the stress of being in debt hovering over your head. Stress clogs arteries, raises blood pressure, causes heart attacks, and basically attacks your entire body. And worrying about getting bills paid, I would have to say, is one of the most stressful things a person can experience in life. Our bodies can handle short term stress, and there's no way around having bouts of small stressful situations in life. You are going to have those moments of stress, like job interviews, business meetings, a new job, a new work task, traffic jams, mother-in-law visit. But those stressors are all short term.

The burden of debt doesn't go away until the debt is paid. So, when you go to look for that new car or that new house, ask yourself – can I safely afford this without causing myself grief and worry in the long run? Because if you can't, it's not worth your health. And, while it may seem exciting and fun at the moment, the excitement will shortly fade, and it won't be as fun if it causes you to worry every day of your life.

I'm not a professional money manager and I don't pretend to be. I do, however, recommend Dave Ramsey's radio show, and maybe some of his books on money management. I listen to his show a lot, and I think he's exhibits a great deal of wisdom in the area of finance that we can all profit from. One of the principles Dave Ramsey hit on repeatedly is don't borrow. Don't do it. Of course, in buying a home you may have to borrow, as most of us do, but borrowing does create a burden that can weigh you down mentally, which will wind up affecting you physically and spiritually.

The Dangers of Going Overboard

I have come to the point in my life where I can see more value in being happy than in being rich. So, while I believe we could all stand to make or save more money, family and health are infinitely more valuable. Master your money. Don't let the money master you. It's a tool used to provide for you and your family. It should never take the place of your family. It is possible to put way too much stress on yourself by worrying about saving money for the future, to the point that you miss out on today.

I'm not saying you have to go blow money to be happy, but I am saying if you have enough so that you don't have to borrow, and have some to put into savings every month, then allow yourself the freedom to be content with that. Even if you can't afford to save money right now, or are in debt as most Americans are, do allow yourself the ability to be content where you are, at least emotionally. Living a stress free life is about making the right decisions going forward and accepting current circumstances with a thankful spirit. It's so easy to go overboard one way or the other.

I think we tend to overcompensate on our finances and so forth, based on what our childhood was like. Some people who had poor families and saw their parents ill equipped at money management might go so far the other way that they never enjoy the money they have no matter how much they make. They scrimp and save every dime they've ever earned. Others, who had parents who saved every dime, grow up wanting to spend every dime they earn. We would all do better in life by discerning what is right in our lives, financially or in the realm of healthy living, and not making our decisions based on emotions.

The Bible says that the love of money is the root of all evil, but some people misinterpret that verse entirely. It's not money that is the root of all evil. It's not a sin to make money. It's the love of money. Money is not God. It's not a person either. It's a tool. What do you do with tools? You use them wisely to accomplish goals.

Adrenaline

At some point you have to relax. We need to focus on turning off that constant adrenaline rush of today's fast paced world that was originally meant to get us moving only when a danger was present. Adrenaline, or stress, comes into our bodies when we need that extra push to get things done, but today many have that adrenaline turned on all the time, which doesn't let you sleep at night. Lack of sleep only adds to stress and poor health.

The Bible teaches us to have faith and trust in God for everything, even though work is still necessary to put food on the table. God gives us the opportunity and the strength to work. We need an attitude toward work, and life in general, that avoids the constant state of worry and panic most of us suffer from today. Our bodies can adapt to normal every day work stress, but we need to have some down time to keep a balance in our lives. We need times where we can free our minds of stress and activity, if we want to be healthy and live as long as God intends for us to on this earth. I believe God gives us a choice in this world. If you want to live on high octane and worry yourself to death, God will let you. So don't be surprised when you hit the pearly gates and St. Peter asks," What are you doing here so early?"

I'm all for looking forward and meeting goals, obviously, but when concern and motivation to make our lives better crosses over to worry and obsession, it becomes an unhealthy burden. It's a fine line, but one a person has to be careful to maintain if they want to realize an optimum healthy lifestyle.

We have the ability to be content or not content, to a certain extent. I'm sure you know people who have very little and seem to be happy, and people that have huge amounts in the bank, but are very unhappy. I know people that practically drive away their family and friends because of their obsession over money, definitely an unhealthy balance.

Make goals, and allow yourself to be content on the way to the goal whether it's financial or physical. Remember, by reaching for a goal, even if you miss it, you are still farther along than before you aimed for that target, whatever it may be.

I notice some people out there, especially some teenagers, lack any motivation whatsoever and create a different kind of stress for themselves. We are created by God to have purpose. We need goals and objectives to achieve or the result more often than not is depression. A person without purpose is more likely to feel depressed. Depression is a form of stress which again we all know is bad on the body. That's another reason exercise is great. If nothing else it gives you a goal and a purpose with which to fill your extra time. The fact that it's healthy in general, on top of that, is just a win-win situation. Of course, most of us, if anything, complain about not having enough time to exercise, but that's another issue altogether. The next time you see your kids lying around like vegetables in their room, you might actually make them happier if you give them something to do. Of course, they would never admit to it, but once they get started, they may actually smile.

Remember that the quest for health isn't just about a number on a scale. A healthy lifestyle starts with your attitude. Being happy and content makes a huge difference in a person's health as compared to a lifestyle of worry and stress. People who would never dream of lighting a cigarette will worry themselves to death faster than a pack a day smoker can smoke themselves to death.

Marathons Are Not Necessary

Some studies are now showing that marathoners may actually be harming their health by causing scarring of the heart. Exercise has been proven again and again to be beneficial to our health, but apparently we weren't meant to go 20+ miles at a time without rest. Some doctors are recommending short bouts of high intensity once to twice a week to build muscle and cardio more efficiently than long slow runs. Personally, I like to go for a balance. Some people will do only one kind of exercise and that's it, but I love to do as many different varieties as possible, like weight lifting, sprinting, jogging on occasion, basketball, and just walking around the park with my wife. I rarely go jogging for more than five or so miles at a time, though. In fact, it's rare that I go more than two miles at a time. I much prefer to sprint and or walk than jogging.

By looking at athletes, you can get a good idea of what results each activity will produce. Take a look at your average marathoner. They usually are very thin with little muscle. Some professional marathoners look almost like they are starving to death. Compare that to the average sprinter who usually possesses very lean, healthy muscle definition. On the other extreme, the power lifter tends to be very large and muscular, but sometimes carries excess fat as well. The body builder is both muscular and has very little body fat because they focus a lot more on diet than power lifters, who are only concerned with the lifting itself. It's been my personal goal to work on as many areas of fitness as I can squeeze into a week without overtraining. Sometimes, however, a person only has two or three times a week to exercise, which is much better than not doing anything at all. In fact, depending on how much time you sit on your job, and how intense your workouts are, it may be just the right amount.

Here's something else to keep in mind about marathon running. According to a study regular exercise reduces cardiovascular risk by a factor of two or three. But the extended vigorous exercise performed during a marathon raises cardiac risk by seven-fold. That really defeats the purpose of running in the first place.

If you do choose to sprint, I wouldn't just jump right into it. Many people will pull a leg muscle on their first attempt at sprinting. It's something you need to build up to over time.

Sleep

A large majority of Americans these days are not getting enough sleep. There are some disagreements about exactly how much sleep we need every night, but most agree it's around eight hours a night. Being tired all the time is not just bad on your health, it is also dangerous. The National Highway Traffic Safety Administration estimates that drowsy driving results in 1,550 deaths, 71,000 injuries and more than 100,000 accidents each year. That's good enough reason alone to get more sleep. You owe it not only to yourself, but the other people you might pass on the road every day.

It is estimated that people tend to eat 300 more calories a day when they become sleep deprived. Studies have found that the less sleep we get, the more body fat we accumulate. One problem is we seem to crave sweet foods like ice cream when we get tired.

So getting a good night's sleep is imperative to any weight loss plan. In order to do that on a regular basis, if possible, a person should try to go to sleep at about the same time every night, and wake up at about the same time in the morning. It's rough on those that work at night to get adequate sleep. Our sleep cycles work best for our bodies when it's as dark as possible. This helps our bodies create the melatonin that makes us sleep well. So keep it dark in your bedroom. Even light coming from your alarm clock can keep you from sleeping as deeply.

There are some major issues studies have shown that can occur in those that don't get enough sleep at night. Being sleep deprived can weaken your immune system, increase your risk of heart disease, give you stomach ulcers, raise your blood pressure, cause constipation, increase the risk of diseases like cancer, harm your brain, and make you age faster.

So go to bed and get some sleep. Your body will thank you.

Pets Relieve Stress

> Proverbs 12:10
> A righteous man regardeth the life of his beast: but the tender mercies of the wicked are cruel.

Studies show that pets relieve stress. Owning a pet can lower blood pressure, and has been shown to improve the health of people who have suffered a heart attack. I saw a television newscast just the other day that claimed that just watching old re-runs of Lassie could relieve stress.

What is it about pets that makes us calm down? Well most likely, at least with dogs, it's their unconditional love and devotion to the pet owner that makes us relax. You don't have to worry about what you say around a pet; they never argue with you. Having a dog can make you feel more secure and feel less likely to get robbed.

Cats are great too, but don't expect a cat to be devoted to you as much as the cat expects you to be wholly devoted to it.

From personal experience, the best way to enjoy the benefits of stress relief by owning a pet is not to get more pets than you can handle. Just like children, your pet needs lots of attention, and if you don't have time to devote to a pet, it can get very unruly and wind up creating more stress than it relieves. The more time you spend with a pet the more it relaxes you, and the more the pet becomes a well behaved member of the family. It can take a while for new pets and their owners to get in sync, so patience is key.

12 TOP DO'S AND DON'TS HEALTH LIST

The following list is just a way to help you keep in mind the most important things in keeping fit. It's easy to sidetracked in this busy world, so when you need a quick refresher just turn to this page.

Top Health To Do List

1. Eat healthy

We all know what that means, but just to make sure. Eat your vegetables and fruits. Eat nuts and lean meats. Also drink lots of water and tea. Eat organic as much as you can afford.

2. Sleep 8 hours each night

When it comes to being healthy, you have to get a good night's sleep every night. In fact, as we all know, if you don't sleep at all, eventually you will die, just like not eating any food or drinking any water will kill you. Lack of sleep can affect your memory and even impair your ability to drive making it more likely you will have an accident, something that is definitely not healthy. A good night's sleep is vital for muscle recovery after a good workout.

3. Exercise

Exercise relieves stress, which is the top consideration on our "Do Not" list. Living a healthy life must include exercise. You can be skinny without it given a good enough diet, but without it you'll never be as healthy as you could be. Do a variety of exercises that includes cardio and weight training. Weight lifting is a good way to build fat burning muscle and maintain bone density.

4. Vitamin D

Get a few minutes of sun every day, during the middle of the day, to get your daily vitamin D requirements. In the winter, consider taking vitamin D supplements and eat as many foods containing vitamin D as possible such as mushrooms, eggs, sardines, salmon, mackerel, and yogurt. One note, it is possible to get too much vitamin D in supplement form, but impossible to get too much from food or sunlight. Be aware, cod liver oil is sometimes taken for its vitamin D, but it may have excessive amounts of vitamin A, which can make it toxic.

5. Take omega-3 fatty acid

Fish oil supplements are good for the brain, skin, and heart. Omega-3's reduce inflammation throughout the body. It does the exact opposite of what sugar does to the body. These days, you have to be really careful how much fish you eat due to mercury content. Wild caught salmon is about the best you can do in terms of getting omega-3's in real food. Tuna should be eaten sparingly. It has been found to have more mercury, depending on where it's caught and what species is used in the particular brand you buy.

6. Go to church and pray

Studies have shown that prayer and regular church attendance go hand in hand with a longer, healthier life.

7. Be consistent

Exercise, eat healthy, and do all the things on this list as part of your regular routine. Temporary diets never work. It's how you live from day to day, every day, that makes you fit and healthy.

8. Beware of man-made food

When in doubt, eat natural. You can't do any better than eating real food. The more man messes around with food, the worse it gets. If you can get the nutrients you need in food, then skip the supplement. The one exception may be fish oil.

9. Avoid using food for fun

This is just my own personal opinion here. I'm not saying you shouldn't enjoy eating, but don't put food up there as the only thing you know to do to have fun. Find other things you enjoy doing besides eating. Go play outside. Do things. Build things. Go bike riding, swimming, hiking, or pass a ball or Frisbee. Have fun, and try to eat to live, and not live to eat!

10. Eat organic whenever possible

I know sometimes it's difficult to be able to spend the extra money on organic food, but for some produce, like apples, it really is imperative that you buy organic. Check out the list in the organic section in Chapter 8 for the clean and dirty lists to determine which produce has more pesticides than others.

Top Health Don't List

1. Do not stress

We'll talk a lot more in detail about this throughout the book, but it's important to realize that controlling stress and worry in your life is the most important thing you can do for your health. Personally, I believe this is a spiritual issue as much as it is a physical one. Being content with the state you find yourself in goes a long way to living longer too. A person's emotional state controls the physical state a person finds themselves in later down the road, and can result in immediate changes to their body as well.

2. Do not smoke

I think we all know smoking is the single worst habit you can find yourself doing. If you want to live a healthy life smoking has got to go, no ifs, ands, or buts about it.

3. Do not eat sugary processed foods

Sugar is as bad, or nearly as bad as smoking. Thanks to the high sugar content in today's average diet. the world is becoming super-sized and diabetes is on the rise like never before. Surely no one could argue that, to at least some extent, sugar is as bad as or worse than any drug on the market. Don't believe me when I say sugar is addictive? Ask yourself if you are feeling angry and defensive over even the thought of giving up your sugary meals, and then tell me it's not addictive. Those addicted to sugar feel defensive about any persuasion to give it up, much like smokers and drug addicts.

Remember fruits have lots of sugar, but they also contain lots of vitamins and fiber. Be aware it is possible to overdo eating fruit thanks to the sugar, but for people who crave something sweet, replacing processed sugary foods with fruits is a great place to start. Add vegetables to the mix and your days of being addicted to sugar are surely numbered.

4. Do not diet

Before you even start a "diet" you should consider what you plan on eating once the diet is finished. If you go right back eating the same foods as before, you will just gain back all the weight you lost and then some. Special diets are a waste of time. It's what you what you eat and drink on a regular basis you need to worry about. Change your lifestyle, change your life.

5. Do not drink diet drinks

Studies have shown that those who drink diet will, in many cases, gain even more fat than those drinking regular sugary drinks. It's just not healthy. Replace soft drinks with healthy tea or just plain water with lemon or lime juice squeezed in. Replacing soft drinks is a great way to shed pounds over a year's time.

13 DRUG CONSIDERATIONS

Don't get me wrong, from some of the things you are about to read, modern medicine has greatly increased the length and quality of life in America and in the rest of the world. Modern medicine is definitely something to thank God for every day, but I think as a whole, society is putting more emphasis on treating problems with drugs after the fact rather than seeking to avoid health issues from the start with healthier lifestyle choices.

Drugs shouldn't be the first thing we turn to for every little ache and pain, or every time we feel a bit down. Drugs are serious business and have too many possible serious side effects to be taken lightly.

I recently read that, according to recent statistics, the average American senior is on more than 31 medications. Elvis Presley only had fourteen different prescription medications present in his body when he died. It would seem logical to assume that 31 medications should be considered a little much for seniors, at least on average.

We do not take the risks associated with taking prescription drugs seriously enough. At the time, Elvis was said to not feel as though he was taking anything wrong because the drugs were prescribed by a doctor. Just because a doctor signs off on a medication doesn't mean there are no potential side effects. There are risks involved with every drug available. We tend to overlook those risks and not take the time to look over the lists of possible side effects as advised by our pharmacists and doctors.

A person should know exactly what they are putting into their bodies at all times. That's why they give you warning labels, because even the safest drug in the world is dangerous if you take too much. Read the warnings and do research about all prescriptions you take. Know what the side effects are and if there are any alternative treatments. If you have doubts about your doctor's advice, then get a second opinion.

You or someone you know may be taking drugs to control diabetes, even after being told by their doctor that it could be controlled by eating properly and exercising. Some folks would actually rather take drugs than give up their junk food. Of course, if you have a condition that can't be managed any other way, then thank God for the medicine.

Drug Companies in the News

Recently in the news, one of the world's drug giants plead guilty and was fined up to $3 billion to resolve federal criminal and civil inquiries from the illegal promotion of its products. Some of the complaints the company was charged with were promoting one drug for treating depression in children without FDA approval and promoting another drug for weight loss, sexual dysfunction, substance addictions, and attention deficit hyperactivity disorder when the drug was only approved for treatment of major depressive disorder.

This news has brought to light some of the big drug company practices of promoting drugs to doctors for uses that are not approved. One of the world's biggest drug makers was accused of encouraging doctors to prescribe its drugs in exchange for free golf, massages, and junkets to posh resorts.

With the occurrence of illegally promoting drugs for uses not authorized by the FDA, can we feel safe that what we are being prescribed medications based on the evidence of the drug's effectiveness and not on that particular drug's promotion campaign?

I'm certainly not saying you should go against your doctor's advice, but common sense dictates that we have to take the ultimate responsibility for what goes into our bodies. Research everything your doctor prescribes, and if you have reason to doubt get a second opinion. Take time to read the warnings that come with every prescription and make sure you fully understand them.

These days people go to the doctor asking for and sometimes even demanding drugs for everything when a lifestyle change would work better and have much healthier long term results. We've become addicted to quick fixes, and are not willing to think long term anymore. Changing to a healthier lifestyle can eventually make it possible for a person's doctor to take someone off a prescription drug, in many cases, further down the road.

The overprescribing of antidepressants for depression is of great concern today. Antidepressants have a variety of possible side effects and shouldn't be handed out to just anyone that is going through a down time in their lives.

Despite the recent recession, Americans have more material possessions than at any other time in history. Yet we seem to be more depressed than ever. First though, let's admit something, it really isn't feasible to have a completely pain free existence or one without any sort of depression. Drugs change the chemical makeup of the brain, and some drugs might cause some permanent physical changes to the mind, causing addiction or other mental illness.

It's not that we can say drugs should never be used in extreme cases of depression or mental illness, but we must ask ourselves – do the drugs work, and are the risks worth it? Most antidepressants come with warnings of possible side effects that include worsening depression and the possibility of creating suicidal thoughts within the patient. As a possible result, some believe that an increase in the number of prescriptions for antidepressants given to service men and women has also increased the suicide rate in the military. There have been a record number of suicides in the military in the last decade.

One study reported that patients who had attempted suicide were more likely to have received antidepressants than patients who did not attempt suicide.

Ask your doctor if there are more natural steps you can take to help in cases of depression. Perhaps, your doctor might recommend something as simple as taking walks every evening, or changing your diet, which could make a huge difference in your outlook on life.

Famous Christians Who Suffered Depression

We can't ignore the fact that some of the greatest Christians of all time have had problems with depression. Look at King David and some of what he wrote in the Psalms. Elijah was depressed and hid away from the world.

> In 1 Kings 19:4-5 referring to Elijah -
> 4 But he himself went a day's journey into the wilderness, and came and sat down under a juniper tree: and he requested for himself that he might die; and said, It is enough; now, O LORD, take away my life; for I am not better than my fathers. 5 And as he lay and slept under a juniper tree, behold, then an angel touched him, and said unto him, Arise and eat.

Of course, Job was depressed after losing everything he owned in life.

In Matthew 26: 38 Jesus said in the garden of Gethsemane, "My soul is exceeding sorrowful, even unto death: tarry ye here, and watch with me."

If even Jesus, our Lord, can feel sorrow, then maybe we should not rush to drugs for help when things look or feel bad. There are times in life when we are going to feel sorrow and times of lengthy depression, but we can always turn to Jesus for help. He knows our sorrows and understands our pain.

Famous ministers like Martin Luther and Charles Spurgeon suffered from depression. In 1527 Martin Luther wrote: "For more than a week I was close to the gates of death and hell. I trembled in all my members. Christ was wholly lost." According to Luther's famous biographer, Roland Bainton, Luther found himself "subject to recurrent periods of exaltation and depression of spirit." Luther himself had written that "the content of the depressions was always the same, the loss of faith that God is good and that He is good to me." Charles Spurgeon actually missed being in his pulpit for two to three months a year because of his depression.

Natural Ways to Combat Depression

One of the best ways to help in fighting any negative physical condition is to take proactive steps before it happens. If you start to feel depressed ask yourself if there are physical reasons for it. Here are some things to consider.

Omega-3 fats, like you find in good old fish oil, have been thought to improve feelings of depression. Omega-3 fats increase blood flow to the brain, and may affect the levels and functioning of both serotonin and dopamine in the brain.

Exercise as well has shown to work well to create positive emotions in people. Eating well and exercising properly while avoiding stress and getting a good night's sleep can help the average person feel better about themselves.

Get some sunshine. One of the reasons we can get depressed is not getting outside enough. We need sunshine to make vitamin D which is essential for healthy living. Hanging out in dark areas for too long can make you feel very down and depressed. Just being in a well lit room can bring some level of increased happiness. Spend time outside every day. There really isn't any better source of vitamin D than sunlight exposure. Lite skinned people need about ten minutes or so a day to get a daily dose of vitamin D. Any more than and the body can't process it. Darker skinned people may take up to an hour outside every day to get a full dose of vitamin D from the sun. Any more than that and you should wear more clothing, hats, sunglasses etc. to protect from too much sun and skin cancer. I could go on forever about the multitude of benefits now thought to be associated with good vitamin D levels, which include lowering the risk of cancer and lots of other diseases.

Play tennis, walk around the park, go outside and play with your dog. All these simple types of activity can make a person feel better about life.

Addressing a person's spiritual and emotional needs is essential in battling depression. Whatever happened to just leaning on Jesus? Prayer and quite time in Bible study can make a huge difference in a person's life.

We can control how we feel up to a point by what we think about. Thinking on inspirational and encouraging scriptures can help when we are depressed and discouraged.

Philippians 4:8
Finally, brethren, whatsoever things are true, whatsoever things are honest, whatsoever things are just, whatsoever things are pure, whatsoever things are lovely, whatsoever things are of good report; if there be any virtue, and if there be any praise, think on these things.

Counting your blessings is another great way to feel better.

Hebrews 13:5
5 Let your conversation be without covetousness; and be content with such things as ye have: for he hath said, I will never leave thee, nor forsake thee.

We are going to have to deal with some depression in life. Just like stress itself, I think we need to think of addressing the management of depression verses trying to completely eliminate it from our lives. Being proactive toward living a healthy lifestyle before depression, or other illnesses, set in is the best medicine.

Overuse of Antibiotics

It actually may be dangerous to take too many antibiotics because over time a person may develop drug resistance. Today doctors are being urged to limit antibiotic prescriptions to avoid the development of antibiotic resistant diseases. The scariest scenario I can think of is to become infected with something that does not respond to antibiotics.

Not only we do have to concern ourselves with being prescribed too many antibiotics, but we have to consider all the meat we eat that has been injected with antibiotics. Part of the reason livestock from any particular farm may get pumped with antibiotics may have to do with how filthy their living conditions are. Some farms use antibiotics just to avoid spending more money on better conditions for the livestock. Stressed animals from poor living conditions are often not fit to eat. So I encourage you to buy foods that come from animals that aren't given hormones or antibiotics. Not only does help protect you and your family from coming down with an antibiotic resistant infection, you also potentially get meat that is much healthier and cleaner.

To avoid the cycle of overuse of antibiotics for common ills, do the simple stuff I discuss all through this book. Eat healthy, exercise, and pay attention to how you feel before you get sick. Be proactive.

For instance, if you feel like you might be coming down with something, try chicken soup for colds, and to help fight infections try eating garlic. Garlic is a natural way to fight bacteria. Any time I feel like I may be coming down with something, or if I think I might have some kind of sinus infection coming on, I go for the garlic and it cures me almost every time within a day. The trick is to get to it just as soon as you feel something coming on. Do not underestimate the power of garlic. The smell is worth the results it brings.

A little extra vitamin C and zinc never hurts either when you feel a cold coming. Good dietary sources of zinc are meats, fish, and beans. A good way to get a natural boost of vitamin C is to squeeze some lemon and lime juice into a glass of water, and make a drink out of it. You can add some stevia for flavor.

Again, the trick is to notice your symptoms early and start taking steps to fight a cold or flu the moment you feel it coming on. But even if you come down with something, go ahead and take the extra vitamin c, zinc, and garlic. The only warning about garlic is if you suffer from heartburn you might want to test some small amounts first.

Always crush garlic and put it in food, like soup, or on a sandwich. In my own experiences, the more you mix it with food, the less heartburn I find you have to deal with.

Wash your hands before eating is one I think we all have down pat, hopefully. If anything, we probably wash our hands too much to the point it dries out our skin which makes it easier for germs to get through the skin barrier.

It's a good idea to get away from anti-bacterial soaps and hand sanitizers and stick to the regular soap, as some say that anti-bacterial products can lead to superbugs.

If individuals don't take the time and effort to make their lifestyles healthier, we may find more and more that modern medicine is just not enough to combat every illness that comes our way as new drug resistant bacteria is created in our pursuit of destroying all bacteria in the world. It's time we all use the wisdom of Solomon and plan ahead before we find ourselves sick and hurting.

Is Hair Worth It?

Here's a great example of why we need to think carefully about what prescriptions we take. I was reading an article the other day that described a terrible ordeal a man was facing in his life because he took a particular drug for hair loss. According to the news article, the thirty year old was prescribed the drug by his doctor. It took from May 2011 until October of that year for him to become completely impotent. The man slipped into a mental fog and even after he stopped taking the drug the ill effects still did not go away.

Another twenty-nine year old man reported suffering anxiety and crippling depression, and claims his doctor never warned him of any possible side effects when he was prescribed the drug. He went on to be declared unfit for duty at his job with the Department of Homeland Security in Texas.

Some drugs given for hair loss work by blocking the conversion of testosterone into a more potent form, called DHT, which contributes to hair loss. Some reports claim that the same effect can be had by taking natural supplements like Saw Palmetto, which hasn't had any major side effects reported. The article I read didn't say precisely, but the side effects described by these and other men seem to indicate an almost complete loss of testosterone. Testosterone is essential not only for sex, but is also responsible for feelings of drive and ambition as well as building muscle.

Before taking any drug, we need to ask if the benefits of a particular drug worth the risks? If the disease is life threatening or debilitating the answer would probably be yes in most cases, but what about for lesser issues like hair loss or other cosmetic problems?

Pain Medications

Again it's prudent to consider the side effects of any drug you take even if it's over the counter medication. Even though aspirin is recommended by a lot of doctors to decrease risks of heart attack, it comes with its own risks, like an increased risk of stomach ulcers and may break down muscle tissue.

Acetaminophen is harmful to the liver and some reports suggest it to be one of the leading causes of liver damage.

Many times simple supplements like fish oil and avoiding inflammation causing sugar can do a lot towards relieving mild pain much more safely and just as effectively as pain medications.

Make sure you have a doctor that is willing to take the time to go over all the side effects and risks involved with any treatment they may offer you. It's never wrong to ask for a second opinion.

The bottom line is, if there is a natural solution to avoid getting sick in the first place, that is, by diet or nutrition, then shouldn't that be our first choice over any other means of care. Prevention, logically should always come first in treating illnesses, if at all possible.

14 MOTIVATION AND INSPIRATION

Everyone is motivated by different ideas, concepts, and events in their lives. The trick to getting on track to a healthy fit lifestyle is finding those things that motivate you, and then mapping out goals for yourself.

I hope that everyone that reads this book will have at least come to the conclusion that eating real food and ditching processed sugary junk food has become their number one health goal. Everything really hinges on a person's diet, and making it healthy should be our first goal, even over and above exercise, as important as that is to a healthy body.

Of course, by writing to Christians I already assume that the primary goal of your life is to walk closely to Christ, which is the most important part of a Christian's life. Without a close walk with God nothing else works in a Christian's life.

There are many inspirational health and fitness examples out there that a person can use to get motivated, whether it's a fitness guru, or your favorite actor, but one of the biggest motivational factors should start with the basics. We need to be in shape so we can be around as long as possible for our families and be a blessing to others. We need to be healthy so we can have the energy we need to do what we have to do on a daily basis to make a living and take care of our families. It takes energy, and energy doesn't just come from caffeine. Real lasting energy comes from a sensible healthy lifestyle based on a good diet and exercise program.

Fit for Marriage

Marriage isn't the ok signal to lie down and die. I think too often we take our spouses for granted. There's definitely nothing wrong with wanting to look good for your spouse. Being fit and trim, and filled with more energy could really add a lot of zest and energy to a couple's relationship. One thing is for sure, an early grave doesn't do a lot for a marriage. Obesity and being out of shape in general is going to take the fun out of your years, and the years out of your fun in marriage.

Simply getting rid of soft drinks, pizzas, fried chicken, hot dogs, and white bread, and replacing them with water, teas, fruits, vegetables, lean chicken breast without the breading, whole wheat bread, etc. can add up to several pounds of fat loss in a year without adding that much more physical activity. Add to it muscle gain by just working out thirty minutes a day, or an hour every other day, can work miracles. It just takes a little patience and a little perseverance to adapt to the change.

We weren't made to eat garbage. If we were, then our bodies would look better the more processed sugary food we ate. It doesn't take nearly as much effort to lose weight once you realize that the junk you eat isn't food, and you begin to realize what real food is. What's more valuable, a piece of cake, or looking good for the one you love? The bakery may want to argue this point, but then they make money off your appetite for sugar.

For Your Kids

The best way to help our kids and the next generation is to be a good example for them. Show them what a good meal looks like, and the results of an active lifestyle. Helping make yourself healthy and fit goes a long way toward making your kids healthy in their own lifestyles.

It's Fun

Being fit is fun! Think of all the fun things you can do when you have the physical capacity. Eating healthy and exercising can help you perform physical activities later in life. Everyone has different activities they can enjoy, whether it's baseball, basketball, golf, horse shoes, Frisbee, gardening, or just walking at the park. It's hard to enjoy anything when you feel bad, or feel like you have no energy from all the junk food and lack of exercise. If you are saving for retirement think about what kind of retirement it's going to be. Are you going to be stuck on the couch the rest of your life, or are you going to be able to get out and do things? If you are already retired, don't you want to stay active or become more active to enjoy the years God has given you?

Movie Inspirations

Growing up in my early teens I watched the series of Rocky movies, starring Sylvester Stallone, over and over again. Back then, Stallone was considered the ideal athlete for the 1980's. Even today, a few decades later, Stallone is still in great shape and still cranking out action movies. One of the things I find so motivational about those movies is the spirit of Rocky Balboa, portrayed by Stallone, which was one of never ending determination. Of course, a few times Rocky gets into the dumps, like we all do, until his wife Adrian gives him a few words of encouragement. Then it's back to training like no man has trained before with Rocky's super motivational theme in the background.

Once in the ring, Rocky would keep fighting, never giving in, even when faced with a much bigger, stronger, and more powerful challenger. If Rocky got knocked down, he would just get up again and again until he won. Growing up a little on the smaller side, I found that very encouraging. In fact, the idea that a man can work hard enough that he can take on any challenge is something I think Americans need more than ever these days. It's part of the American spirit to take on challenges and overcome them with hard work and a never say die attitude.

This goes along with a Biblical principle found in Proverbs 24:16: For a just man falleth seven times, and riseth up again: but the wicked shall fall into mischief.

Today Americans are losing their will to fight. Obesity is taking over, and people would rather sit all day than pick up a weight or even go for a walk. The great thing about the Rocky movies is the attitude Rocky displays of never quitting no matter what. Wouldn't it be nice to see people getting off their couches and heading out to the parks to play some kind of sports, just any kind?

The food today has just drained men and women of the will to do anything. If it's not the sugar, it's the chemicals, antibiotics, fat, and everything else they can cram into our lunches, that messes with weight and testosterone levels making girls go through puberty faster and giving men attributes more like women. The chemical additives in our foods today make it harder and harder for both women and men to lose weight.

On top of that society hasn't exactly been progressing toward a more competitive edge. More and more it seems like winning is considered mean spirited. In a man, if you take away the chance for success, that is, to win, you take away the whole reason to get involved in the first place. We are made to compete, but these days competition, even in business is getting a bum rap. These days kids are given awards just for showing up to a game.

What can you do? Well besides cutting out processed foods, you should aim to eat as many organic foods as possible, and get out and exercise, whether you want to or not. It's time we stop babying ourselves and get up.

Rocky never would have won a fight if he waited for government assistance. He sure never would have won if he ate junk food all day, and he most definitely would never have won if he sat on the couch feeling sorry for himself.

Somebody reading this is going to say that's just a movie. Sure but then take a look at any successful boxer or athlete. Do you think winning comes easy? Just as Rocky says in the movie, it takes heart. It takes strong will and determination sometimes just to take that first step toward a healthy lifestyle, but I guarantee that the more you get out and do things, the better you will feel. For the more advanced athlete the lesson is to keep pushing for the next level.

One thing or another is going to happen if you keep trying and failing in a fitness program. You are either going to get real mad and quit, or get real mad and keep going harder than you did before. You never lose as long as you keep playing the game. The second you quit for good then it's over, but like the Bible says, the righteous falls and gets up again and again.

Those of us that work out all the time may be tempted to give up if we don't quite see the results we want as fast as we want. Don't quit. Just get mad and work harder. Think smarter about how you approach your workouts and what foods you eat. It's all about experimenting. Be careful though to avoid the pitfall of overtraining because that lessons your ability to work out at your full capacity and just slows down your progress. It could also lead to injury, so always remember to work out smart as much as you work out hard.

Most of the time it's your diet you need to address first. Intensity in a workout needs to be added to slowly but surely, or you risk getting hurt.

So when you look in the mirror and you don't like what you see, don't blame the government, society, your spouse, or the guy next door. Get mad at yourself and do something about it. Notice I said you do something about it. Getting mad and down on yourself without action is useless and self-destructive. Use your emotions for a positive instead of a negative. The tendency we have today to blame everyone but the one that has any control over our situation, namely ourselves, is pointless and self-defeating.

If you hit a roadblock with your fitness goals, start from scratch. Write down everything you eat. Is there anything that should go? Are you getting enough rest, or enough sunshine during the week to keep your vitamin D levels up. Maybe you need to start upping the intensity of your workouts, or just changing them around to shock your body. If you keep working on it you'll figure it out.

For women especially, you don't need any special starvation diets that kill muscle and slow down your metabolism. All they do is leave you in worse shape than when you started. Getting fit is a lifestyle. It happens gradually over time, or it doesn't work.

One of the best scenes from any of the Rocky movies was on the last movie in 2006. Rocky's son tries to discourage Rocky from fighting due to his advanced age, but Rocky has a different take on it. Rocky tells his son, and I'm paraphrasing here, that nobody hits as hard as life, but that what makes the difference is moving forward no matter how hard you get hit. That's how you win in the end, by always moving forward.

That pretty much sums up life. You either take what life throws at you and keep going, or you quit. But for all those thinking about giving up, you have to ask yourself, where does giving up leave you? Once you give up, whether it's fitness or something else, what you are really giving up when you quit trying is hope. As long as you keep putting forth the effort, you always have that hope of getting to where you want to be in life. Moving forward is the only way to not only achieve goals, but also to keep your hope and happiness alive.

Personal responsibility has been replaced by people wanting others to do everything for them, and when it comes to your health nobody can do for you. I think the reason so many people are becoming overweight these days is because the mentality of society is to demand your rights and privileges, but there are some things, like health, you can't demand from the government, or anybody else. Sure, healthcare is important, but even the best healthcare system in the world won't help a man who sits all day and constantly puts poisonous junk food into his body.

Don't get me wrong, there are things the government should do, like requiring that genetically modified foods be labeled so we know what type of food we are getting. We the people need to make the decisions as to what we eat or don't eat, but the government should assist us in having all the facts, especially in this day and age where what you see isn't always what you get. I'm not big on government regulations. They always wind up making things worse than when they started, but simply making sure food gets labeled properly as to what type it is and how it was prepared is a great way to assist Americans in making healthy choices.

Another great concept where Rocky is concerned is that going one more round when you don't think you can makes all the difference. It's true. The reason diets and exercise plans fail is because people quit way too soon. As I've said before, diet plans are worthless to begin with. What a person who is serious about getting and staying healthy should do is develop a diet lifestyle transformation and stick to it. The nice thing about your taste buds is that once you start to give them healthy food long enough, they'll start to appreciate the taste of healthy foods. You'll actually begin to love the taste of healthy natural food.

Exercise isn't something you start one day and finish the next. It's something you have to keep doing over and over again on a consistent basis throughout your entire life. So find the kind of exercises you enjoy or can at least live with. Besides, for you couch potatoes out there, sitting on the couch all day everyday has got to get boring after a while, right?

Achieving goals makes workouts more fun. Really putting yourself into a workout not only causes you get better results, but it makes working out a whole lot more interesting. So set goals in the areas where you want to the most results. Do you want bigger arms? Then set a goal of lifting more in curls. Do you want to be more ripped? Then set a goal of sprinting faster for a 100 yards. Make your athletic goals fit your physical goals. For those just starting out, do something you enjoy and you will work out without boredom and wind up hooked on exercise instead of chocolate chip cookies.

I think after watching Rocky III for the millionth time, this scene has stuck in my mind. Rocky was feeling really down and his training was off, so he wanted to put off training until tomorrow. Apollo Creed, who trained Rocky in this movie, replied back angrily, "There is no tomorrow!" In a sense, when it comes to getting fit, there really isn't a tomorrow. Too many people postpone eating healthy and exercising until it's too late. Don't wait until you get sick to start working out and eating right. Do it before you get sick.

Jack Lalanne

Everyone who is really into working out and staying in shape owes a bit of gratitude to the godfather of fitness, Jack Lalanne. Jack Lalanne invented a number of exercise machines, including the leg-extension and pulley devices.

Jack Lalanne started where much of America is right now, addicted to sugar. He described himself as being a "sugarholic" and a "junk food junkie" until he was fifteen, claiming his addiction to sugar had given him behavioral problems. After listening to a public lecture by Paul Bragg, a well-known nutrition speaker, Lalanne began his obsession with fitness and nutrition.

In the 1950's, Lalanne started one of the most popular and long lasting fitness shows of all time. The show lasted from 1951 to 1985. Before there was high fructose corn syrup, he was preaching against sugar dependence on his TV program in the 1950's, comparing people that were addicted to sugar to alcoholics.

Jack's father died of a heart attack at the early age of 58, while he lived to be 96 years old.

I'm sure there are some things that Lalanne advocated that may have been disproven by today's modern science, but he definitely steered fitness in the right direction. He preached against processed foods and made good nutrition one of his primary focuses to having a fit body. He always worked out for two hours a day, although studies today recommend only thirty minutes to an hour a day, but, then again, it's unlikely that anybody working out only an hour a day could match Jack Lalanne's physical feats of strength. A popular story goes that Arnold Schwarzenegger himself was beaten by Jack Lalanne in a push-up and pull-up contest when Arnold was 21 and Jack was 54 years old.

Watching old clips of Jack Lalanne taught me how to make great healthy desserts. While mine might differ a little from what he proposed, one of my favorites, inspired by Jack, consists of low fat yogurt, unsweetened coconut, blueberries, nuts, and a banana all mixed together. It tastes as good as ice cream. Jack's version consisted of a smashed banana on a plate, raisins, just a little coconut, and a little honey.

Make Goals and Find Motivated Friends

Most of us know that we tend to pick up habits and lifestyles of our friends. This trend really kicks into high gear in high school and continues to a lesser degree as we get older. If your spouse has bad habits, it's more difficult for you to set good ones. But, on the positive side, once you do improve your habits, you can use that to your advantage and be a great motivating force for your spouse.

Find some people in the gym to workout with that are stronger, faster, and generally fitter than you are. It's the best way to get motivated. The personalities of those you hang with are going to influence your personality traits given enough time. We tend to copy people without even realizing it. Think of this – if your friends are always eating junk food and smoking in front of you, how long will it be before at least one of their bad habits becomes your own? Not to mention the bad health effects of second hand smoke. It is very difficult to avoid eating junk food if it's constantly waved in your face. By contrast, people motivated for health and fitness will pull you their way, and competing with friends in the gym is definitely a great way to make you push yourself harder. Just don't go overboard and kill yourself trying to lift the same weight your bud has been lifting for years in just a matter of days.

Listen to your favorite music while exercising. This always helps me, and there have been studies to show that when people listen to their favorite tunes, they will push harder and longer, and go farther in endurance exercises than those who didn't listen to music. On the way home after a big workout, you might want to stick in some relaxing music, but while working out, personally, I like fast paced music to really keep me going.

Create goals. Creating goals is essential if a person is going to succeed. You have to know what you're aiming at before you start shooting or you are not going to hit anything. Our pastor likes to say something to the effect that if you aim your arrow at a hard target a long way off, your arrow will fly much farther than if you aim it straight to the ground. I believe that to be true. Aim high. Setting big goals for yourself can put you a lot further ahead in life than looking at the ground and moping ever will. The trick is to have big goals for the long term and smaller goals for the short term to help encourage you along the way.

Don't be afraid to dream big because dreams are where motivation lies. You can always tell when someone has lost the ability to dream, or imagine themselves achieving goals or bettering their lives. They have that terrible defeated look on their faces. See yourself succeeding, Imagine it and feel it. I guarantee you that almost every highly successful person, especially in the area of sports or fitness, saw themselves at some point achieving a goal or a dream long before they ever did. If you don't believe you can do it, you never will. It's not about being unrealistic; it's about allowing yourself to see the possibility that you can achieve great things. Without hope there is no such thing as motivation. Hopes are founded on dreams and goals for your life. If you reach one goal, set another one.

15 FASTING, IS IT HEALTHY?

The Bible encourages fasting, but stops short of commanding it. Here are a few verses from the Bible regarding the subject of fasting:

Nehemiah 9:1
Now in the twenty and fourth day of this month the children of Israel were assembled with fasting, and with sackclothes, and earth upon them.

Daniel 9:3
And I set my face unto the Lord God, to seek by prayer and supplications, with fasting, and sackcloth, and ashes:

Matthew 17:20-21
20 And Jesus said unto them, Because of your unbelief: for verily I say unto you, If ye have faith as a grain of mustard seed, ye shall say unto this mountain, Remove hence to yonder place; and it shall remove; and nothing shall be impossible unto you. 21 Howbeit this kind goeth not out but by prayer and fasting.

Fasting has become popular of late for reasons other than the spiritual. Some promote fasting for weight loss and even helping to increase longevity. For that reason, much debate has occurred as to what the health effects of fasting really are. There are many arguments for and against fasting as a means for weight loss. Those who believe in the health benefits of fasting claim it increases longevity and refer to animal studies to support their assertion. Some of the other benefits of fasting may include normalizing insulin sensitivity, promoting human growth hormone, lowering triglyceride levels, and reducing inflammation. It is also thought to increase a person's ability to process nutrients from food.

Going without food from 6 to 8 hours is thought to cause the body to start to burn off its fat reserves.

If eating small frequent meals increases metabolism, wouldn't fasting slow metabolism down? My thoughts are that as long as one didn't fast daily, their metabolism shouldn't be significantly affected. An example would be skipping breakfast every day.

Those that support fasting as a health regime suggest you can lose fat and still build muscle even if you fast frequently. This does seem to ignore the concept of muscle wasting whereby the body tends to devour muscle first before going to fat reserves. This is why body builders tend to eat much more frequently so as to avoid muscle loss.

Keep in mind that what a person eats once the fast is over is important, especially if the fast lasts over 8 hours. Rushing to a fast food joint and pigging out after fasting, will likely ruin any health gains attained during the fast. You will see the best results if you eat real food after a fast.

I think it's also important to keep in mind that the body will adapt to your regular eating schedule. If you normally eat every three hours and then add one fasting day per week in which you skip one to three meals, the effects are likely to be more positive towards weight loss and fat burning than if you fast every day. Fasting too often would most likely result in muscle loss; something to keep in mind for those focused on muscle building. The body will adapt to fewer calories after a while, and slow down the metabolism as a result.

A person that skips breakfast every day and then begins eating breakfast again later may see some weight gain at first because of the additional calories consumed; however, I would not discourage someone from adding breakfast to their daily meals if they have traditionally skipped breakfast. Studies have shown that those that eat breakfast are more likely to lose fat than those that skip breakfast. Eventually, after eating a healthy breakfast daily, the body would likely adjust itself and the breakfast meals would aid the person in losing weight over the long term when combined with muscle building exercise. The key, of course, to staying healthy and losing fat, as always, is determining the most healthy habits that you can live with and sticking to them.

Those that oppose fasting for weight loss say that fasting can be dangerous for those who have not been on a healthy diet, and it distracts from the more efficient weight loss plan of eating several small healthy meals during the day. People who should not fast are pregnant women, people with wasting diseases, malnutrition, history of cardiac arrhythmias, or hepatic insufficiency. It is not recommended to take Tylenol during a fast, and those with liver or kidney issues should be careful about fasting.

Those are some of the issues to consider before fasting. Hopefully, this information can be helpful to you whether you are considering fasting for spiritual or health reasons.

Certainly Jesus would not have mentioned fasting as a means to answered prayer unless fasting was a good thing both spiritually and physically, but it is a good idea to be careful and put a lot of thought into fasting, especially if you haven't fasted in the past. For the time being, the pros and cons of fasting are heavily debated among the medical community, and may well be for some time to come. Personally, I wouldn't fast just for weight loss, but always being health conscious, I think it's a great idea to be aware of the potential effects on the body, both good and bad, during a fast. Always, when in doubt see a doctor first before trying anything new.

16 IS ALCOHOL HEALTHY OR DEADLY?

Many people believe the occasional use of alcohol isn't a problem. You've probably even read recent news stories suggesting that having a beer or a glass of wine a day is actually good for your cardiovascular system.

If your goal is to live a longer, healthier life, we have to look at more than just the reports of cardiovascular health benefits. We need to look at the bigger picture and also weigh all of the negatives of drinking alcohol. Some doctors say that the health benefits of alcohol lie more in the probable socialization that follows with social drinking rather than the alcohol itself. So the reports of health benefits of alcohol aren't exactly concrete.

One of the health benefits of going to church is said to be gained from the social aspects. Human beings are healthier in general when they interact with others. Alcohol is certainly not necessary to achieve socialization. It just happens to follow some instances of socialization.

So what about the negative health effects of alcohol? Unfortunately, they are numerous indeed. Granted, most of the health risks associated with alcohol are related to overuse, but any use increases the risk of diseases, and the risk of becoming addicted to alcohol, which opens the door wide for all kinds of problems. Even with moderate alcohol intake, there are increased risks of injuries, violence, certain forms of cancer, liver disease and hypertension.

The psychiatric disorders associated with alcoholism include major depression, dysthymia, mania, hypomania, panic disorder, phobias, generalized anxiety disorder, personality disorders, schizophrenia, suicide, brain damage, neurological deficits, which include impairments of working memory, emotions, executive functions, visuospatial abilities, and balance.

Alcoholism may cause coronary heart disease, ischemic stroke, and cancers of the respiratory system, digestive system, liver, breast and ovaries. Alcoholism also accelerates the aging process.

Every time you take a drink, you have to be aware that you are taking a chance. No one ever became an alcoholic that didn't first take a drink.

Consider what alcohol does to your belly too. Alcohol contains seven calories per gram, which is more than carbohydrates and protein, but with no nutritional value. The liver will metabolize alcohol first over fat, which is most likely because alcohol is seen by the body as a toxin. Drinking alcohol increases fat around the internal organs, which is definitely not a healthy place for it to be.

And, while beer commercials may imply that only the manliest of men drink beer, remember that alcohol decreases testosterone production for up to 24 hours after you've had that drink. Testosterone is vital in creating muscle and, thus, lowering fat. On top of that, beer also encourages estrogen production, which compounds the decrease in testosterone. So the next time you see tough guys drinking beer on TV, remember, they may not be feeling so manly on the inside. Maybe that's why men are often seen crying in their beer when they get drunk. It's probably due to all the extra emotional sensitivity they are likely experiencing.

Drinking alcohol may even make the drinker insulin resistant the same way drinking cokes and eating too much sugar does. So when all of the health effects of alcohol are weighed together, alcohol just doesn't belong in health conscious person's lifestyle.

So what does the Bible say about the subject of drinking alcohol?

Proverbs 20:1
Wine is a mocker, strong drink is raging: and whosoever is deceived thereby is not wise.

Habakkuk 2:15
Woe unto him that giveth his neighbour drink, that puttest thy bottle to him, and makest him drunken also, that thou mayest look on their nakedness!

Isaiah 5:11
Woe unto them that rise up early in the morning, that they may follow strong drink; that continue until night, till wine inflame them!

Isaiah 5:22
Woe unto them that are mighty to drink wine, and men of strength to mingle strong drink:

But...didn't Jesus make wine for a wedding party?

John 4:46
So Jesus came again into Cana of Galilee, where he made the water wine.

The New Testament, translated from Greek, uses the word "wine" for both fermented and unfermented drink. After reading previous scriptures condemning strong drink, it doesn't seem logical that Jesus would make alcoholic wine for a party. Knowing how many things God has created for us that are healthy to eat, I don't believe Jesus would have created alcoholic wine that could destroy a person's liver, or possibly tempt someone into getting drunk. God never tempts anyone to sin, and even a liberal view of wine is negative in regard to getting drunk. It just doesn't follow logic that Jesus would put anybody into that kind of situation.

Further, as we've discussed, alcohol is a toxin to the body. Would Jesus offer a toxin to others? Would God warn of the dangers of strong drink and then offer it to others? So it would seem that the most logical conclusion is that Jesus created a non-alcoholic grape juice.

Inevitably, we have to conclude from the many problems associated with alcohol that the dangers and risks outweigh any perceived health benefits.

17 GOD'S ETERNAL LIFE HEALTH PLAN

Throughout this book we've examined a lot of common sense health principles that were backed up by God's word way before modern science ever existed to confirm these ideas with studies and research.

God has given us so many things to promote health, from the foods He created, to the mechanisms of exercise, that if we stopped right there, we would have so much to be thankful for, but God has also provided a way to beat death entirely. Sure, everyone dies physically in this world, but the Bible teaches us that there is more to our existence than what we experience here on Earth. The Bible teaches that human beings have souls, and where the soul goes after death depends on the awesome gift of salvation that can be obtained through Jesus Christ alone.

Jesus is the only way to heaven after we die. Only by trusting in him, and him alone, can a person have assurance that heaven is their eternal destination, where sickness and death are a thing of the past. It's not how good you are, or what you've done or not done. It's simply a matter of accepting Jesus and what He did on the cross as payment for your sins.

Romans 3:23
For all have sinned, and come short of the glory of God;

We've all broken God's laws one way or the other. We all are guilty. To God sin is a serious matter.

Just imagine getting into heaven like someone wanting to come into your home that had been wallowing in a mud hole. Imagine them sitting down on your sofa and chairs and tracking mud into your home. You probably wouldn't like that. To God wallowing in sin is much worse than mud. He made a way to cleanse us from our sin through the blood of Jesus Christ, shed on Calvary's cross.

Revelation 1:5
And from Jesus Christ, who is the faithful witness, and the first begotten of the dead, and the prince of the kings of the earth. Unto him that loved us, and washed us from our sins in his own blood,

To be washed from our sins just takes trusting Jesus as Lord and Savior resting upon his death at Calvary as payment in full for every sin you've ever committed or will commit. That makes you clean and acceptable by God to enter into heaven.

It's all summed up perfectly in this simple but powerful verse:

John 3:16
For God so loved the world, that he gave his only begotten Son, that whosoever believeth in him should not perish, but have everlasting life.

You can't find a better health plan than that.

ABOUT THE AUTHOR

Tim Frady has been an avid body builder for over 25 years, and is the webmaster of the health and fitness news site http://hip2bfit.com, and as such, keeps abreast of all the latest health news and information. Most importantly, he has been a born again Christian since he was a child in kindergarten and believes that the Bible is the infallible Word of God.

www.ingramcontent.com/pod-product-compliance
Lightning Source LLC
Chambersburg PA
CBHW070119010626
45794CB00012B/290